This book would be informative to those interested in the following subjects:

Tai Chi, Chi Kung, meditation, energetic healing, out of body experiences, remote viewing, afterlife explorations, pyschokinetics, relationships and love.

The IMMORTAL'S GIFT

A Parable for the Soul

Vincent J. Lasorso, Jr.

Layout & Design – Kevin Pease

Publisher's Cataloging-in-Publication
Lasorso, Vincent J.
     The immortal's gift : a parable for the soul/
Vincent J. Lasorso, Jr. -- 1st ed.
     p. cm.
     LCCN: 00-132151
     ISBN: 0-9679867-1-0

     1. Taoism--Fiction. 2. T'ai chi ch'uan--
Fiction. 3. Spiritual life--Taoism--Fiction.
4. Taoists--Fiction. I. Title

PS3562.A7755I46 2000   813.6
               QBI00-398

This book is dedicated to my fairy wife Connie,
who taught my heart to fly.

ACKNOWLEDGEMENTS

This book is a product of my life experiences. Therefore, everyone who has ever been in contact with me, or with persons in contact with me, needs to be thanked and acknowledged. Somehow, you the reader, influenced the creation of this book. Everyone in this world is inter-related and inter-connected. So, thank you for your contribution. However, there are certain persons whose influence in this project deserve special acknowledgement and thanks. First the masters who gave me first hand instruction and experience in the magic of the internal arts: The Immortals, Grandmaster Lu Hung-Ping, Mufundishi Nganga Tolo-naa, Robert A. Monroe, Master Tanka Ramos, Grandmaster Peter Robinson. Next there was Nancy Revere Todd, whose work and support inspired me to write this book, and Helen Meines, whose initial editing prevented much embarrassment. Then there was Jody Robinson and the fine folks at Millennium Marketing whose expertise and insights brought the book into its final form. But very special thanks goes to editor Jim Fogt, whose talents, insights, and inner guidance, brought out the best of this story and its characters. Jim is a master in his own write. And through it all, there was my dear wife and best friend, Connie, whose love, support, tolerance and teaching is the reason this book exists.

AUTHORS PREFACE

Students have asked me for years, to recommend a good book on Tai Chi. This was never an easy task since the majority of Tai Chi books are about Tai Chi Chuan, the physical martial art that Tai Chi students practice to obtain Tai Chi.

Tai Chi Chuan books follow the same general format: Twenty pages dedicated to: a history of the art; a history of the particular style; a history of the author and their lineage; the health and mental benefits. The next fifty pages are dedicated to "how to do our style" techniques. Then there is a chapter about the "advanced benefits/techniques" and martial arts applications. Tai Chi Chuan books are basically "do it yourself" technical manuals that quote the scriptures of Tao Te Ching and the classics of the ancient masters.

Real Tai Chi, on the other hand, is the harmony of Yin: the nonphysical forces and energies of existence, with the Yang: physical forces and energies of existence. This balance is obtained by physically exercising the mind/body through Chi Kung and forms, and the mind/spirit through meditation and spiritual explorations. The mind determines the success of this balance. The mind is where Tai Chi exists.

A good book about Tai Chi is a book about the mind. How the mind works, how the mind creates balance, and how the mind utilizes the processes of Tai Chi Chuan and meditation to create a balanced fulfilled life. This was not an easy task. My previous attempts accomplished the task, but were boring, heady, works that were not easily understood. I was perplexed. Then a good friend of mine, Nancy Revere Todd, asked for my opinion of her manuscript. I read the manuscript of her novel *Virgins* and thought to myself, "I wish I could write good fiction." I thought about the possibilities of writing a fiction and realized I had nothing to write about. Four months later, I simply sat down with my laptop, and started writing this book. It literally just appeared. As I progressed it was clear that I was writing the "Tai Chi" book I had attempted before as an entertaining parable. In thirty days, the story was complete. All the concepts I had tried so hard to express, were revealed through the turbulent life and colorful adventures of a 13th Century Chinese Taoist Monk. Our hero is not one of those dumb characters of most "spiritual unfolding" novels. When we meet Hunglu, he is already an accomplished priest, warrior, artist, and healer. Thus, the reader has the opportunity to discover new methods of meditation, healing and physical techniques as they travel and explore both sides of existence through the eyes of an experienced teacher.

Learning and understanding unfolds with time, so when I wrote this book it was important to write a story that would always have meaning. The reader does not have to understand the concepts and experiences to enjoy the story. Enjoying the story, our story, is the lesson.

Vincent J. Lasorso, Jr.
December, 1999

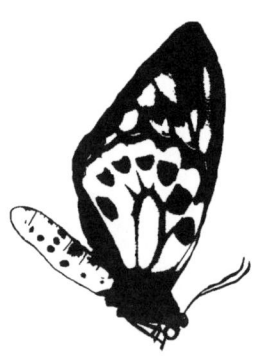

THE PARROT

Rudely awakened from his meditation under a mountain pine bough, a man dressed in the airy silks of a Taoist monk bolted upright and frantically looked from side to side. He slid his fingers over one ear, locking his thin black hair behind it, then cocked his head sideways. Again the monk heard the piercing screech that first roused him from his peace. Ten feet in front of him and strutting out of the brush was a peacock. It stared at the monk with deep, expressionless eyes, then fanned its tail feathers.

"You silly thing!" Hunglu yelled.

The peacock turned its head, pinpointing him with its gaze. Its ruffling feathers refracted warm afternoon sunlight, creating a magnificent display of color.

"You want a nut, don't you? Lazy bird!" Hunglu smiled, reached into his belt pouch, and pulled out a fresh pine nut as the bird crouched forward with an open mouth. Having secured its meal, the peacock happily wandered off.

This was an innocent encounter, but one that would mark the moment Hunglu embarked on his greatest journey. He would never forget waking up on that cool mountaintop, the shrill cry of the peacock calling him out of his dreams and into a greater awareness of himself and the world around him.

Hunglu was a man who long struggled to answer life's many questions. He knew that the peacock may have been a divine sign or simply another visit from one of his many feathered friends—in either case, one had to be open to the possibilities. His fellow monks said that the birds recognized Hunglu as one of their own because of his acquired skill in astral travel. His gift of spiritual flight and affinity with avian beings earned Hunglu the name of Flying Spirit.

He had spent the last seven years in a monastery, training in the spiritual, martial, and healing arts. Now, at thirty-six years old, Hunglu had traveled through space and time and had gone beyond the veil of death. He performed seemingly impossible feats in physical reality, learned to employ the healing herbs and exercises of Chinese medicine, mastered the art of warfare, and even designed and supervised the construction of many building projects. Hunglu's experiences were extensive, but unfortunately some had been costly to his body, mind, and soul. Down Hunglu's back lay bundled striations of raised, purplish skin. These marks were the remains of a great violence from his past. Few people around him knew of the scars, for Hunglu did not wear them with pride. Nor did he share his stories easily with others. For this reason, he was considered one of the best listeners among the monks, but the truth was that Hunglu did not know if the monks with whom he lived could be made to understand his past.

Thinking about the day he earned his battle marks was not easy, and actually talking about the scars seemed an impossibility. From time to time, he could feel the wounds of his past ignite recollections of battles long since fought. In those moments, Hunglu tended to hurry off to his private quarters, desperate to descend into a tranquillity exercise. Deep meditation was the only reprieve from the fiery sensation spreading across his back.

Healing was slow and required enormous patience, but Hunglu's life was now mostly peaceful. He had taken on the role of counselor, helping students resolve conflicts between their meditations and their lives—a position usually reserved for much older monks. It was a great honor the Grandmaster of the temple had bestowed on him. In his counseling sessions, Hunglu found that the answers to questions posed by his students were already within them; he needed only to wait and listen and the newest monks would come to their own conclusions. His was an occupation filled with rewards.

His transition from warrior to counselor had not been easy, though. He had known many tragedies as well as triumphs in both pursuits. Life for Hunglu was an endless quest to understand himself and others, and he was aware that he could more effectively perform his counseling duties only *after* he resolved some of his own issues.

There were occasions when Hunglu felt as if he were close to finding his spiritual self, but those moments were rare. Mostly he wondered if he would *ever* locate his true inner-self. And if he did, what would he find?

Hunglu kept these confused feelings to himself—like so many people in the world. He was afraid to express his doubts, afraid of what others might think of him, especially those whom he counseled. Though he had been a hero in war, a disciple of the greatest Taoist philosophers and healers, and a well-respected member of his monastery, Hunglu was still alone, without family, without a sense of home. In tense moments, he fell into private meditations, where he felt most safe. And when his loneliness was at its greatest intensity, meditation was the only thing Hunglu could do to keep himself from grabbing one of his fellow monks and shouting out, *Why am I here?*

Yet, after completing his mental and physical exercises, Hunglu always emerged cleansed, at peace for a time. Extreme shifts in emotion had become so commonplace to him that Hunglu suspected the constant alternating between tranquility and chaos was the way *all* humans lived.

From his life in the monastery, Hunglu realized that each monk had a unique temperament and family conditioning from the past. But the discipline of a monastic life restrained them from indulging in negative personality patterns and continually presented opportunities to shed limiting social habits and behaviors. The goal of monastic training was to recapture the Being of the Uncarved Block, to rediscover a mind not sculpted by social forces, and uncover the pure nature of the individual. Towards this end, Hunglu had done everything the spiritual classics extolled. He was mostly proud and happy with his life since coming to the monastery. Then he met the Butterfly Immortal. And that was when the *real* questions began.

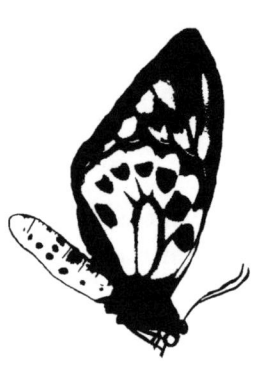

HOLDING THE BALL

The Butterfly Immortal first appeared to Hunglu in dreams. He was considered by the Taoists to be the ancient sage Chang Tzu. In the dreams, Hunglu found himself upon the mountain where the Butterfly Immortal and his disciples trained and instructed him. He could not see these beings except as bright splashes of light moving quickly about. However, Hunglu could hear them talking to him through his mind and body. More importantly, Hunglu could *feel* them surrounding him. It was a wonderful sensation, remarkably calming to his soul.

From the Butterfly Immortal, Hunglu learned secrets of Taoist philosophy and martial arts, far more than he could have gleaned through ordinary monastic studies. This education had been going on for two years, during which time Hunglu continually brought the knowledge he was acquiring to the temple's Grandmaster. The Grandmaster was a dark-eyed man whose tiny body was splintered with wrinkles. Despite his serious appearance, inside the Grandmaster was a soul filled with compassion and wisdom. Hunglu trusted him as a friend and as a surrogate father.

Hunglu continually asked the Grandmaster to explain what was happening and *who* was teaching him, but the Grandmaster told the young monk not to be concerned about such questions, to observe and practice what he was being taught. Above all, he urged Hunglu to be patient; time would reveal true understanding.

Despite the sense that something of great importance was happening to him, Hunglu went on in his daily life, engaging in the routines of a good Taoist monk: meditation, prayer, work, and exercises for the body and spirit.

One of Hunglu's favorite practices was a meditation called Holding the Ball. Holding the Ball required Hunglu to stand with his knees bent and his arms held at shoulder height, similar to sitting on a horse. With the palms of his hands facing inward, as if grasping a large ball, the posture replicated a tree standing in the universe, gathering energy and releasing resistance. Considered the bridge to explorative meditation, it allowed Hunglu to travel to distant realms of consciousness, blending perceptions of the nonphysical Yin side of life with the physical Yang side. He routinely did this practice for an hour before his Tai Chi exercises. It was on the day he met his peacock friend that Hunglu had decided to enhance his usual day's practice with an extra-long session of Holding the Ball.

Not long after he settled into the standing posture Hunglu became relaxed and was overcome with a peace to which he was not accustomed. Slowly, the trees and sky blurred and the physical world started to dissolve around him until, finally, he was able to focus and move toward a mountain. Deep in his meditative state, Hunglu found himself standing before the Butterfly Immortal and quickly tried to compose himself; he was, after all, the Flying Spirit. These experiences, though not unusual for him, were nonetheless surprising. This time, though, he sensed things were different . . . this was *really* happening! Everything in his heart and mind told him so.

"I have chosen you to be one of my disciples," a familiar voice said. "For years I have taught you in your dreams. But now you have reached the level of immortality where your dreams are real. This, Hunglu, is what you sense here."

"You have spent many years learning to explore the realities within your dreams and meditations. You have mastered the techniques to enter into these realities at will. But now . . . now you must learn about your own world. In your efforts to explore the Yin side of life you have forgotten the Yang. You must study the physical world and your humanness to find the true secrets of immortality and perfection."

"Butterfly Immortal—" Hunglu began. There were so many questions he wanted to ask. But there was no answer, just a sensation of the ground dropping out from under his feet, the world spinning gently, and a feeling that he was quickly descending to another reality. Then, suddenly, he was beneath the mountain pine bough again.

Though slightly dazed from his rapid transition between realities, Hunglu became aware of a screeching sound coming from nearby bushes—this time it was not the peacock. Recognizing the frantic notes of a smaller bird in distress, Hunglu put his encounter with the Butterfly Immortal aside and hurried over to the bushes. The monk approached very cautiously as his senses cleared. He did not want to frighten the bird. Parting the bushes, he found the source of the cry: a fledgling parrot.

"Poor little one, where is your mother?" Hunglu asked soothingly.

The bird screeched again, then lapsed into frozen silence.

A scan of the surrounding area revealed blue feathers and the remains of the mother. It was clear she was a victim of a predator who had found the parrot nest in a tree hole. In the ensuing battle for life, the fledging must have fallen out of the nest and survived only by hiding in the underbrush.

At this age, the parrot would not be able to feed itself or fly. Its hunger made it cry out for food to a mother no longer capable of meeting its needs. It was clear to Hunglu that certain death awaited the poor bird.

He looked into the young bird's black eyes and spoke gently: "Little one, do not be afraid. *I* will take care of you."

The parrot cocked its head, screeched, and ran into the thickets. The suddenness of the gesture startled Hunglu. What am I getting into, he wondered. There was an air of uncertain prophecy that lay just beyond Hunglu's ability to understand, but without hesitation he reached into the brush after the bird. Carefully, he picked up the fragile creature and began stroking it until it became complacent.

"I think I'm getting into more work than I can imagine," Hunglu murmured as he closely inspected the bird for the first time. He could feel the tiny bite of its claws nervously constricting against his palm. It was a sad little thing, and Hunglu knew that it only consented to his touch because it no longer had any alternatives.

The baby parrot was a very rare bird for that part of China, and even more so for its coloring. It was a blue parrot with a black ring around its neck. Hunglu had heard of such birds from farther south, but other than peacocks he had never seen a bird of this color. He had no idea how it came to this location, but he did know he would have to care for it if the parrot was going to survive. First, he would need to find it some food.

Hunglu placed the parrot gently in his belt pouch. A quick look into the nest gave him some clues as to what the bird ate, and the monk went about gathering the right nuts and berries while the bird slept comfortably against his belly.

Feeling the almost imperceptible weight of the tiny life in his pouch, Hunglu found himself remembering what it felt like to lose a mother at a young age. He suddenly could not help reflecting sadly upon his own experiences. Recalling his past sometimes left Hunglu feeling as if his present life was falling apart. "How did I get here?" Hunglu whispered aloud with confusion in both his heart and mind. *Am I insane?* he wondered.

Though the image of the Butterfly Immortal was burned into his being, the mundane task of gathering berries and the unexpected sadness in his heart made him question what had transpired in his meditative state. Had the Butterfly Immortal really advised him to explore reality? Why *should* he explore the physical world with all of its pain and suffering? Why not exist purely on the spiritual plane?

He felt himself grow frustrated, not because of the Butterfly Immortal's command, but because the question of reality had always been difficult for Hunglu. It seemed he never knew where he belonged—the spiritual world, the physical plane, *somewhere in between?* It had been this way all his life, ever since the well. *The well!*

A highly charged moment from his past, everything Hunglu had ever accomplished always came back to the well. It was the memory that for so many years consumed him.

THE WELL

It was the middle of autumn in his fourth year when Hunglu sneaked away from his mother's attention and out to the village well to get a drink of water. The villagers shared a thin stone well that filled superbly in the wet season, yet the water was always several feet from the top of the hole. This made it easy for adults to drink from, but children were not permitted near it. They were made to drink from a bucket brought up specifically for them when there were no adults around. The bucket water tasted of sour wood oil and grew hot sitting in the sun all morning. The well water, on the other hand, was cool and sweet. With no apparent witnesses, the choice was clear to Hunglu.

It was the middle part of the day, when most of the men were tending to crops and most of the women were inside preparing the noon meal. Young Hunglu glanced around, then climbed up the hot stones and knelt by the shadowy edge. Reaching over with a cupped hand, he stretched and leaned and then, with a shriek of surprise, he lost his balance and violently pitched forward.

When Hunglu's head hit the cold water, the shock immediately stopped his breathing. As he submerged, his body twisted, rubbing against the slick stone walls. Frantically, he tried to push himself out of the well, but his hands simply slipped along the surface. Hunglu turned his head to face upward, but his feet were above him and there was not enough room to curl his body and turn around. He was trapped facedown in the water.

Helplessly, the child looked up at the unreachable air, his gaze piercing the clear blue sky and reaching into eternity. Dying was not so bad when he came to accept it. Yes, Hunglu realized, he was going to die, but it did not feel tragic or scary to him now. Time passed slowly and the last of the air in his lungs gave way to silvery bubbles. Hunglu sank into a peaceful unconsciousness.

Suddenly he felt his body jumping out of the water and into the sky. Cool, clean air filled him, and the young boy gasped as he raced upward toward the clouds. The sky turned into a bright light. He felt an incredible love and warmth that made him feel safe. In the distance a bird flew toward him—a blue bird . . .

By falling so deeply into his past, already Hunglu had ignored the Butterfly Immortal's command to explore the real world. Gently pinching a blackberry, he admonished himself, but Hunglu knew that the key to his life was somewhere in his recollection of past events. He looked down at the little blue parrot, safe and warm in his belt pouch. Saving the tiny bird's life should be his focus, but he found himself remembering his mother's embrace at the side of the well.

Yes, his mother snatched him from death and gave him life again. Hunglu recalled how the process of dying in the well was bittersweet. There was fear and loneliness—yet something glorious lay beyond. That had been the beginning of his avian gift, his astral travels, his spiritual quest, and his unexplainable longing to find a place for himself among the immortals. Yet, how could he come to this place? What was the path?

With his hands cupped and filled with colorful nuts and berries, Hunglu and the parrot returned to a small one-room cabin he had built in the woods at the southern edge of the temple complex. The Grandmaster had granted him special permission to construct private quarters outside the complex, enabling Hunglu to be free of disturbances while he explored the dreams and teachings of the Butterfly Immortal. Here Hunglu would try to do as the Butterfly Immortal instructed. He would attempt to explore his Yang.

In the cabin, Hunglu carried the bird's food to a bowl in front of his prayer altar. He poured the nuts and berries into it and, using a river stone, ground the ingredients into a lavender paste. He added water and some extra grain to make a cold porridge. The activity and smells woke the bird, which poked its head out of Hunglu's pouch and started screeching. The parrot stretched its neck, trying to reach the bowl with its yellow beak.

"Are you hungry, little one?" the monk asked. "Then let's see if you will eat for me." Daubing his finger into the food, Hunglu presented it to the small creature. Without hesitation, the bird aggressively took both the food and finger into its mouth, eating until its crop bulged with food. "Well little one, it looks as if we are going to be good friends."

Hunglu smiled at the bird and felt very happy that it so readily took food from him. It made him feel good that he could save this small life. And perhaps he had even found a new friend.

"Now where can we put you, little one?" Hunglu whispered. After some thought, he was able to fashion a nest out of the food bowl and a small woolen blanket. He then placed the blanket-covered bowl upon his bed mat. "I'll be back shortly, little one," he assured the parrot. "I must go to the temple for prayer services now."

Leaving the bird safely behind, Hunglu walked to the temple, following a worn path that was barely illuminated by the setting sun. Thoughts filled his mind as he hurried to the temple: he liked the bird but wondered what the fragile creature's presence meant. The baby parrot had come to him immediately after his vision of the Immortal Butterfly. But it also closely resembled the bird from his near-fatal experience at the well. Hunglu pondered the events of his day but came to no conclusions as he entered the dim temple hall. He attempted to momentarily free his mind of questions, but looking up at the beautiful statue of Quan Yin, the goddess of compassion and healing, he couldn't keep himself from remembering his mother's death.

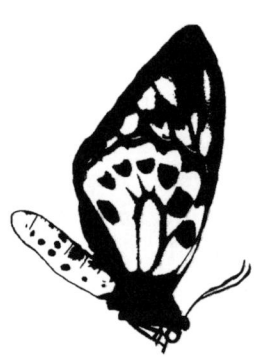

LOSS

Hunglu's mother had wasted away before his eyes. Over a period of six months, she just kept getting weaker and weaker as an unknown illness ravaged her body. The village doctor was helpless to stop the disease's course. Hunglu spent hours watching the doctor use all the tools of his trade—herbs, needles, and massage—to no avail.

During this time Hunglu got to know the doctor, who was a Taoist with his own tragic past. The child blindly trusted the doctor, but even Hunglu could see the doctor growing increasingly distressed by his inability to help Hunglu's mother. One day, after a few months of treatments, the doctor took him aside.

"Child, there are many times when my techniques can provide a small comfort for people, but that is all. You must understand that there are many people beyond any help I can give." Compassionately placing his hand upon Hunglu's shoulder, he went on: "It hurts my heart to tell you this, Hunglu . . . but your mother . . . she is going to die."

The words pierced Hunglu's soul. Only twelve years old, it was inconceivable to him that he would spend the rest of his life without his mother. He was an only child; his mother was his whole life. His father's personality paled next to her luminescent spirit. He was not an unkind man, but Hunglu's mother was the only one who really understood why the boy was different. It was as if she knew his destiny and was grooming him for it. Hunglu sensed that she held the answers to important questions that would come to him soon. She was his guide.

The shocking news nearly overwhelmed Hunglu, but he reasoned that if anyone in the world could answer the single-most-important question burning within his mind, it was the doctor.

"Why is she dying?" Hunglu cried from the depths of his heart.

"Hunglu . . . only the gods know for sure," the doctor answered. "But this is what my experience has led me to believe: among the myriad of creatures, every life has a purpose and a soul to guide that purpose. The purpose can be as common as an insect sacrificing its life for another creature's survival or as grand as a chosen one becoming an emperor. Yet, once its purpose is accomplished, the soul begins to stop the vital life force—*Chi*—from flowing to the body. This is the beginning of the dying process. Death will then release the soul for another purpose. As a physician, I can only help support a life in harmony with the soul's purpose. At times like this I do the best I can to prevent needless suffering."

"Why does the soul do this?" Hunglu asked.

"I really cannot explain it," the doctor said. His voice was kind but sorrowful. "Only an immortal knows and understands the secrets of the soul . . ."

"Then I will find the immortals," Hunglu said defiantly.

"They are in another world," the doctor said. "You must understand that."

"I will travel to it."

"It is not so easy, child."

The doctor was grim, but Hunglu was determined. He began by searching the familiar hills around the village. The sun beat down on Hunglu, scorching his tender flesh. There were no immortals to be found.

The child returned after sundown, his skin burned to a rich red hue.

Hunglu's father, in from the fields, sat sleeping at the side of his mother's bed. Exhausted, the child went to his own bed; he had not been defeated, he had only just begun.

In the end, though, the doctor was correct. Finding his way to the immortal world was not easy for Hunglu: the path was entirely unclear, and the quest consumed him for the next twenty-four years.

Hunglu's mother died that night. The boy woke and felt a cool wind rush into the room. It encircled his burning face, soothing him like a cool hand. Then the breeze simply dissipated and his flesh became like fire. That is when he knew she died.

Hunglu had been his mother's only child. She had one stillbirth and two miscarriages before he was born. Barely surviving Hunglu's birth, she was unable to bear any more children. This was a curse for the family. A rice farmer rarely prospered with only two hands doing the work. But his father, Hungling, was no ordinary rice farmer. Before Hunglu was born Hungling and his wife worked very hard, long days producing rice. While they had no children and were both free to work, they had a great surplus of rice to sell and barter.

Hungling invested in planting root vegetables that required little care, like carrots. Then he planted chestnut and cherry trees. Soon Hungling started selling vegetables and fruits that were unavailable anywhere else in the region. The investment worked. By the time Hunglu was born, his father had established a market and a fortune by growing low-maintenance crops. Hunglu was raised as a farmer's son, heir to the land and wealth it provided. But then his mother died and Hunglu's life seemed over. Within a year, Hungling married the widow Sunyin from the nearby village.

Sunyin was a young mother with four children—three sons and one daughter. Her husband had also died of disease, like Hunglu's mother, and Sunyin was forced to live with her brother, which created a hardship for them all. Without a husband and property, Sunyin's sons had no chance for a future other than servitude. She actively sought out Hungling after his wife's death, offering her services as a maid and her sons as labor for food, lodging, and a hope for her family's future.

Sunyin was an answer to Hungling's household needs and could provide him the means for further success as a result of her drive and ambition. Sunyin was also pretty, with a simple farm-girl's charm. It wasn't long before Sunyin was sharing Hungling's bed as a wife, and ten months later Hunglu had a half-brother.

All of Sunyin's boys were older, stronger, and more experienced workers than Hunglu, and Sunyin took every opportunity to demonstrate the value of her sons to Hungling. But to truly assure her sons' future, she knew she would have to find a way to get Hunglu out of the family. Sunyin argued that Hunglu was not necessary, and suggested he go live with Hungling's brother-in-law in the north. It was not Sunyin's arguments that led Hungling to his decision, though. He could see that the older boys intimidated Hunglu. Hungling's son was introspective, shy, and intellectual. He clearly did not belong on a farm, and Hungling knew that the boy was miserable. Although it broke his heart, under the circumstances Hungling felt it best for Hunglu to leave. So at fourteen years of age Hunglu was sent off to live with his uncle near Nanking. It would not be a bad life for the boy, Hungling knew. The child would grow up in relative luxury, safe to pursue a more genteel style of living.

He did not intend to abandon his son completely, but with Sunyin's boys helping, the farm grew quickly and there was little time for travel or even notes north. In some ways it was easier for Hungling to convince himself that the coarseness of plantation life was better left undiscovered by his son, and he never sent for Hunglu. He believed that Hunglu was somewhere in the northern provinces becoming a great scholar. He could not imagine the boy as anything else.

Hungling would die ten years later, while Hunglu was at war. Hungling never knew the warrior in his son. And Hunglu would lose his inheritance to his stepmother and a half-brother he never knew. It was many months before Hunglu even found out about the death of his father. He took the news stoically, barely allowing himself to feel anything. By then, he was becoming a master at suppressing his emotions. While the grief he felt for the loss of his father was minimal, Hunglu found that profound and painful memories of his mother's death had been unexpectedly resurrected. Throughout his life, he had caught glimpses of his mother in dreams, but never more than that. He had not yet made good on his declaration to find her. He had done many things, learned from many teachers, yet had anything changed?

Hunglu was still alone in one world and unable to find his way to the next. What was *his* purpose? How could he better understand his mission? The encounter with the Butterfly Immortal, the intense *realness* of the experience, made him feel as if something had been put into motion. Still, he was far from the end of his journey. The death of his father seemed to place him even farther back. Why had he never gone to see Hungling in those many years? Hungling was the closest connection to Hunglu's mother, and now it was too late. This error would plague Hunglu for many years.

THE DRAGON

After prayers, Hunglu sought out the Grandmaster in his quarters to tell him about the Butterfly Immortal's most recent visit.

The Grandmaster's room was plain, containing a bed and a small wooden table with two chairs. Outside the window, the calming sounds of night were beginning to settle over the monastery. The Grandmaster sat pensively, yet without a hint of surprise, as Hunglu quietly told the story of his dream.

"I knew this day would come" the Grandmaster said gently. "I will reassign all your responsibilities so you may devote yourself to your new studies."

Hunglu was taken aback by this reaction and felt as if he had done something wrong. Being *released* from duties was akin to being made an outcast.

But the Grandmaster spoke reassuringly: "You are no longer under my jurisdiction. You will now be guided by one of *my* masters."

"One of *your* masters?" Hunglu blurted out.

The Grandmaster laughed at the quizzical look on Hunglu's face. "Of course," he said. "Who did you think counsels and teaches grandmasters?" Then the Grandmaster's expression became more compassionate. "Do not be afraid, Hunglu. You can come to me with your questions and concerns anytime, and I will help you through this."

The words were comforting, yet Hunglu still felt unsure about the changes. The Grandmaster's lifelong counsel and training had greatly changed and influenced the young Taoist's life. The master's role was more that of a father—protecting, guiding, and disciplining the student toward achieving his highest potential. For all this, the formal hierarchy of a master-student relationship was strongly adhered to; without question, it determined one's status within the monastery. But in mere seconds, the Grandmaster had changed Hunglu's status from a disciple to a classmate, as if he had been expecting this all along.

"I understand you have a new friend" the Grandmaster said, suddenly changing the subject.

"Friend?"

Hunglu's confused expression again set a smile to the Grandmaster's ancient face.

"Your blue-feathered friend, Hunglu. I hope it's not too much of a disruption." Patting Hunglu on the shoulder and laughing quietly, the Grandmaster rose from the table and left without further comment.

The one thing Hunglu knew for certain about the Grandmaster was that his laugh always preceded a surprising lesson.

As he walked home from the temple, Hunglu mused about the experience—how did the Grandmaster know about the bird?

It was quiet when Hunglu entered his cabin. The silence amplified his unfounded feelings of impending doom, which quickly found a new focus: *Where was the bird?*

Expecting the worst, he went over to the bowl on his bed and pulled back the blanket, revealing a blue ball, out of which a terrified dark eye looked straight up at him. The parrot screeched loudly then unfolded its blue wings and beat them as if greatly annoyed; it was the sign of a very hungry bird.

Hunglu smiled with relief. He prepared the bird's food and fed it until it was again quiet and content. Then he lay back upon his bed mat, petting the bird and holding it against his chest. Exhausted from the events of the day and soothed by the bird upon his chest, it wasn't long before Hunglu drifted into sleep . . .

There were noises all around him . . . a viewing stand of people dressed in finery watched the warrior . . . a strange beast stood in front of him . . . taunting and snarling! . . . a flurry of motion . . . the beast flashed in front of him . . . a large serpent . . . a dragon . . . rearing upward over thirty feet.

Seasoned from combat and years of training, Hunglu's sword was in his hand before the dragon reached its full height. The olive-colored dragon struck out with its right claw, but Hunglu dove to the ground in front of him, barely evading the strike. Rolling onto his shoulder, Hunglu back-slashed with the under-edge of the blade. The sword cut the tendon below the dragon's thumb, disabling the creature's grasping ability.

Hunglu rolled again before the other claw struck the ground where he lay. In a swift motion, he was on his feet and charged the dragon's underside, twice thrusting his sword into the dragon's chest. He had punctured both of its lungs. Blasts of hot, acrid air nearly forced him to the ground.

The dragon fell forward, but Hunglu leapt sideways to avoid the crushing weight. Then the dragon's body struck the ground with such force that Hunglu's jaw uncontrollably slammed shut. Holding the sword at a menacing angle as he moved down the length of the scaly dragon, Hunglu came to the head of the dragon. He could see his reflection in the moist black ball of the dragon's eye; he could see the warrior within himself.

"You must finish me," the dragon gasped weakly. "Drive your sword through the crown of my head. Do not be slow or too short. Thrust clean and deep."

Hunglu trembled inside at the thought of killing the dragon. This was *murder!* There was no honor in killing a wounded, helpless creature.

"No, I will not kill you!"

"You already have," the dragon roared with great effort. "You must do what is right. False compassion comes from fear, but real compassion comes from the courage to do what is right. Now strike and kill me!"

An adrenaline-saturated heart pounded blood through Hunglu's brain. He quickly climbed to the top of the dragon's head. Every part of him felt sick and resistant to what he was about to do. Struggling slightly to maintain his footing on the slippery hide, he focused on the spot at the crown of the dragon's head. Holding his sword in both hands and using all of his body, he thrust.

The sword pierced the skull easier than Hunglu expected, like punching through a drumhead, but the dragon's brain was as thick as mud, forcing him to push hard to reach the point of death. The sound of bone grinding against his sword hurt his ears . . . his body . . . his soul.

"*Good . . .*" the dragon murmured with his death sigh.

The scene dissolved and reformed around Hunglu as the dragon became the Butterfly Immortal. The spirit was more clear than it had ever been in previous encounters. A face was distinguishable in the bright yellow light—a kind, gentle face.

"People do many things to avoid fear, Hunglu, especially the fear of bad feelings," the Butterfly Immortal said. "They are wise to avoid

19

feelings of guilt, courageous to avoid shame, honorable to avoid loneliness. But people will be motivated by pleasure, too. Rarely do they do what is right for the good of the Tao."

"No matter what you wish others to believe, it is emotion that controls all your decisions and all your actions. As you reflect upon your life, you will discover which emotions direct your life's choices, which ones motivate you, but most importantly, which emotions you avoid. These are the emotions that control your success and create your failings." He smiled knowingly at Hunglu. "To be a master you must know your truth. You must act out of this truth to be in harmony with the workings of your soul and thus be in harmony with the Tao."

Hunglu was about to ask why he was chosen and what he was supposed to do, but a sharp pain ripped through his face, and again his encounter with the Butterfly Immortal was cut short.

He jerked upright from his mat, grabbing at his face, and found the parrot's beak locked onto his mustache.

"Foolish bird!" he yelled as he stripped the parrot from his face and held it in his trembling hands. "Why did I ever take you in?" He was furious at being interrupted by this bird.

The parrot cowered while Hunglu contemplated tossing it out into the woods to fend for itself. He stared at the creature, looking into its eyes . . . and then he calmed. He saw the fear in the bird's eyes . . . fear *he* had caused. The bird had done no wrong. It was only grooming his beard, just as Hunglu had earlier preened its feathers. The bird was acting out of love, out of its truth.

"I'm sorry little one . . . it seems *you* are the master here," Hunglu apologized as he took a pine nut out of his pouch. He mashed it with his teeth and offered it to the bird.

The parrot turned its back to Hunglu.

"I deserved that, little one." He smiled. "You truly are the master here."

The parrot turned back to him, squawked, and took the nut mash, finger and all.

Hunglu pondered the Butterfly Immortal's suggestion that his decisions were governed by emotion. But didn't the Butterfly Immortal understand that he didn't *want* to kill the dragon. Yes, Hunglu resisted. Even though killing was the right action, he had made the *compassionate* choice.

The experience was entirely disconcerting. Hunglu believed that killing wasn't honorable, that it was wrong. Yet in battle he struck mortal blows to the dragon. In the past his mind would have reconciled this action by distinguishing the difference between the need to kill in defense versus killing by choice. But *was* there a difference? His actions in battle and his choice not to kill were both motivated by his fear of death.

Hunglu had killed in battle before. He knew how the survivors suffered their losses of home and family. In war, he reasoned, the dead were the lucky ones.

Still, he knew dying was painful too. This was a pain that came from fear. Survivors feared their future without the presence and love of their dear ones. Those dying feared the unknown, not with their mind but with their heart. The body had a will to survive but, at some point, the body broke down the resolve of the mind, unleashing fear. Hunglu had seen stoic men accept their death, up until the moment before their end, then their minds could no longer check their emotions, and they feared the inevitable.

"Why did people fear so much?" Hunglu wondered as he lay back upon his mat.

The parrot started to snuggle up into his beard.

"Be careful little one," Hunglu warned.

As he fell back into sleep, he knew that there was something he was missing, something he was not seeing.

Rising out of his body . . . floating skyward to the stars . . . watching the stars disappear . . . into another dimension . . . it was as if he was walking inside a cloud, everything around him was cast in shades of white . . . everything he touched felt like love.

In the distance Hunglu saw women talking, and he moved toward them. His movement was neither a walk nor a float, but like a glide. A familiar woman turned toward him. Hunglu recognized her; it was his mother. Her dark hair hung past her shoulder and her rich, brown eyes welcomed him. Hunglu's mother smiled at him and led him to a cool spot beneath a gingko tree.

"My son," she said, "you have struggled so hard with your life. Sit and rest with me for a while."

Hunglu touched the ground beside her and plucked a piece of grass. He felt it, smelled it, tasted it. The colors around him were more vivid and vibrant than normal. *This was real.*

Hunglu knew from his earlier spiritual teachings that everything contained a vital energy. When looking at an object it was not the object he saw, it was its vital energy. But the energy was far different looking through physical eyes than when looking through nonphysical eyes. The Butterfly Immortal had shown him how the difference in perception between these two levels of vision could be explained by looking into a pool of water. The water, like the physical eyes, changed the shapes, colors, and locations of what was seen in the pool. Nonphysical seeing showed one the true image; the intensity and clarity of the vision was a clue that one was in a spiritual dimension. This moment with his mother was so filled with detail that it was too real to be ignored. He could even smell the scent of the sun radiating from her skin.

Hunglu's mother looked at him closely and for a long time. Then she raised her hand and tenderly caressed his cheek. "Love," she suddenly said. "That's what you are missing."

"Love, mother?"

"Yes, Hunglu, you fear the loss of love."

"I don't understand what you mean?"

"That is because you have never allowed yourself to love and to be loved."

"Love causes pain," he said. "It's the cause of all suffering. It is better to avoid those feelings."

She took him in her arms and pulled him near. Hunglu buried his head in her shoulder, closed his eyes, and concentrated on her voice.

"Yes, Hunglu my love, your very protests reveal how important love really is."

Tears welled up in Hunglu's heart. His mother was right.

"The loss of love causes pain," she continued. "It is wise to avoid pain but not love. We avoid love to avoid the pain of loss, and then we suffer pain because we don't choose to love. Hunglu, we can't lose love because it's always with us. Come with me."

She lifted his head. The scene changed and they were no longer beneath the gingko tree. Now they were at the edge of the well, looking down at his drowning four-year-old body.

"Mother, why are we here?" Hunglu asked. There was a deep-rooted fear in his body, an emptiness in the pit of his stomach.

"You need to remember a few things you have forgotten."

"I will love you forever, my son."

She touched his shoulder and he was underwater, drowning. The sudden shift of reality and his inability to breathe pushed Hunglu into a panic. He tried to kick with his feet . . . they wouldn't move . . . nothing would move . . . he was trapped within a frozen body. He screamed inside himself, the silent scream of nightmares, as he submerged into darkness.

Then he was propelled upward at a tremendous speed. This part Hunglu remembered. He soared skyward into a light. The light became a tunnel. As he raced forward, he felt increasing love filling him. Then his body changed into love itself.

From out of the light, a blue bird appeared. Hunglu floated, following the bird. Others were floating all around him. The majority were visions of people that appeared dull, gray, and lifeless. Their limp bodies were scattered about the air and there were so many of them. But there were brighter people too. The brighter ones had a clear, knowing expression and seemed fully aware of where they were and what they were doing. Hunglu noticed that the brighter beings looked less like people and more like tall, oval, white lights. Then he noticed that the bright beings seemed to be teaching and guiding the duller ones. Hunglu watched, trying to comprehend all the activities.

The blue bird circled around the collected light and gray beings, then called out to Hunglu: "Come with me."

Hunglu looked back for his mother. Both she and the tunnel were gone.

Hunglu and the blue bird flew over to a temple with an adjacent courtyard, which was surrounded by cherry trees. There was a reflecting pool and shrine at the north wall. As they flew through the gate Hunglu could see people silently practicing Tai Chi Chuan. The bird perched upon the shoulder of the headmaster who was overlooking the class. Hunglu was surprised to see that the headmaster was the Butterfly Immortal.

"Hello, Flying Spirit," the Butterfly Immortal said. "I am proud of how quickly you are progressing in your lessons." He guided Hunglu around the courtyard, then stopped by the reflecting pool.

Hunglu looked down into the rippling water. His reflection was distorted, yet he could see a vision of himself with absolute clarity.

"You remember the water lesson, Hunglu. Good. Someday, you will build a school like this, but not of mortar and stone. This school is eternal and these students are from many different lifetimes. They come here to learn and share knowledge."

"This is a place that exists between dreams," Hunglu said, awestruck.

The Butterfly Immortal gestured for Hunglu to follow him as he turned toward the center of the courtyard. As they walked, the courtyard dissolved into colored balls of light, floating buoyantly in space. The Butterfly Immortal became radiant, so much so that Hunglu had to turn his eyes away from him. Together they were consumed in light and traveled to a place where Hunglu could see seven other beings of tremendous luminosity around him. They glowed and shimmered like the lights of the night sky.

The seven stars! he thought to himself. He realized he was seeing the celestial masters of guidance referred to heavily in his education at the monastery.

Hunglu was carried to the center of the seven stars. He felt space enwrap him, and he started moving quickly. The love he felt was far more intense than in the previous tunnel through which he passed. He started to sense the thoughts of others, to know things that weren't from his time or his land. He found himself becoming a part of all this knowledge and love, until he no longer existed. Then Hunglu disappeared as a drop of water disappears in a giant sea. He had no sense of his humanness. He was the light, floating outside the circle of the seven stars. They moved in a celestial dance, stopping in a position that resembled a spiral. The pattern of light was instantly burned into him, like an instinct beyond the far reaches of his human origins.

He heard the voice of the Butterfly Immortal: "Hunglu, whenever you need to come here for guidance, remember this pattern in your mind and you will be here with us."

Dream or not, Hunglu was returned to his body. With a tear of joy trickling down his face, he woke to a new morning.

LU AND CHENG

The sun was rising. Hunglu felt a chill from the morning dew filling the air. He wrapped a blanket around his shoulders as he prepared the bird's morning meal. The sun had burned off the dew by the time Hunglu had finished feeding the bird, so he put the small parrot in his belt pouch and walked out to a training area he had prepared. It overlooked a valley and gave Hunglu a sense of place. He put the bird upon a sunlit post and faced the still rising sun.

Standing at attention, evenly balanced and aligned, Hunglu began to breathe, pulling in his lower belly while he inhaled, then relaxing it completely as he exhaled. With each inhalation, he experienced a wave of energy rising from the earth. It coursed through the back of his body to the top of his head. Then he exhaled and the energy flowed down the front of his body into the earth.

He continued by bringing this circulating energy inward, pulling to the core of his body until there was a channel of power pulsing through the center of his body. The pulsating wave became stronger and stronger with each cycle, and when it moved through his core without obstruction, Hunglu began to open each of his seven chakra energy centers.

He concentrated on each center until that region of the body started to relax. One at a time, he imagined a ball of energy forming within each individual region, followed by a sensation of turning. Once he could feel movement, he extended the ball in and out of the body, stimulating the vital energy of that region and energizing the organs it supported. When all centers were opened, he expanded the energy core outward until he was engulfed in one large sphere of energy. He let his physical body melt into the warm sphere as he stood like a tree and moved into the posture of Holding the Ball.

As each moment passed, Hunglu released more physical and mental tension from his body. Soon he could not perceive any physical sensations. He had, by the evidence of his perceptions, become pure energy. It was known that some practitioners of this exercise could literally disappear in front of their disciples. Hunglu himself had stood this way through a rainstorm without a single drop of water touching his body. Now he was ready to move.

Hunglu practiced seven Chi Kung exercises to stretch his body and cultivate energy circulation through all its parts. This was in preparation for a unique Tai Chi form called the Heavenly Dragon. The Heavenly Dragon was a routine of moving into postures possessing more variations in stance and technique than other Tai Chi form sets. Its movements modeled the mythical, physical, and spiritual powers of the dragon. Dragons, magical and immortal beings, were pure energy in physical form. It was believed that imitating the serpentine undulations of the dragon allowed a release of the immortal energy within a human. Hunglu had learned this form from the Grandmaster, and it seemed only appropriate to use it the day after his battle with the Butterfly Immortal disguised as a dragon. The form, though, was not new to Hunglu.

On days when Hunglu felt vigorous and wanted a physical challenge, he practiced this form while stepping upon various-sized posts and stones he had set in the ground. This type of practice developed strength and fine-tuned his physical alignments on uneven terrain—a valuable skill should he have to use these techniques to defend himself. However, today Hunglu simply wanted to let his mind wander, so he chose a smooth piece of ground to practice on. The flow of the movements and energy would help him sort out his experiences and solve some of the problems they had created. As he moved, he reflected upon his life.

Too poor to afford passage north, at fourteen Hunglu made the dangerous three-month journey north with a trader. It was his father's idea. At least Hunglu would have the protection of a group rather than being left to fend for himself on the road. Further, it would not hurt the boy to do physical labor, Hungling thought.

Hunglu worked as a porter, carrying goods on his back for long hours every day. At night his back ached, but he was able to persist. It seemed like safe passage at first, but the caravan was just four days along the road when the first bandits ambushed them.

Dusk had fallen on a winding road, and there was a general weariness from the day's travel. They had been traversing thick woods and the light was dimming quickly. Hunglu's mind was on food and the throbbing in his lower back. The traveling party was by a ford in a stream when the first arrows silently flew through the air, striking the lead horse and rider. Two hired guards in the front were immediately rushed by swordsmen in black flowing robes. As the archer kept the travelers in the middle of the caravan in check, more swordsmen attacked the guards in the rear. The guards were outnumbered two-to-one.

A bearded and fierce-looking guard named Cheng quickly dispatched one attacker by hacking off the bandit's sword arm with a willow-leaf broadsword. The scream of the injured bandit attracted the archer, who drew back on his bow to shoot Cheng. But before the archer could release the arrow, a dagger pierced his biceps and entered his ribcage, pinning his arm to his side. The dagger had been thrown by an unassuming man next to Hunglu. Then the dagger master quickly glided toward the archer and with a fluid movement snapped the enemy's neck. He took up the dead archer's bow and quiver and disappeared into the woods.

Meanwhile, Cheng decapitated a second attacker. The head flopped to the ground near Hunglu, who stood frozen in terror as the lifeless face looked up at him. Cheng rushed to the front of the caravan and quickly killed two more swordsmen, but not before one of the other guards took a mortal blow to the chest.

The remaining front guard had wounded one attacker and was now in a death battle with the second. Both swordsmen were evenly matched, but Cheng wasted no time in taking the bandit's head. To Cheng, a bandit was a rabid dog not deserving of life or honor.

It was over almost as quickly as it had begun. Broken bodies lay strewn about the caravan, blood from mortal wounds draining from the victims into the muddy ruts along the trail.

Moments later, the quiet man came back from the woods with four horses.

"Only four?" complained the trader. "Hardly a fair compensation for the loss of a man and a horse!"

Nothing in his life had prepared Hunglu for this carnage, for this fear, for this wanton disregard for life. The image of Cheng moving behind the bandit swordsman and swinging his blade through the man's neck was almost too much to bear. The bodiless head lived nearly six seconds, the shocked expression on the face of the bandit imprinting a permanent horror on the youth's mind. Hunglu saw the man's dying eyes looking at him for an explanation of his predicament. Then shock and terror took over the face as the bandit began to comprehend his fate. Hunglu watched the bandit's eyes lose their luster as life left them. A moment later he heard Cheng cursing the head: "I will watch wild dogs piss on your head and eat your brains!"

Hunglu turned away and fell down on both knees, quivering.

While Cheng and the others threw the bodies to the side of the road, the quiet man walked over to Hunglu and patted him on the shoulder. "It is safe now, boy."

Hunglu started to sob uncontrollably, putting his face upon the ground, hoping the tears would wash the violent images from his eyes. The quiet man helped him up and took him into the woods. There, Hunglu vomited until he collapsed in a limp, exhausted state.

The man above him spoke: "This is horrible for you, I know. But had things been different we would all be dead right now." The quiet warrior then knelt down beside Hunglu and softly rubbed his back, comforting him. The voice of the man was strong, reassuring. "Listen to me, boy: there is no honor in killing for money. Men like these are consumed by greed and they kill innocent, honest people for money and clothes. But today we killed wolves who prey on lambs, and they will never kill another innocent person again."

The warrior's name was Lu. He had a gentle, pudgy face, though the rest of him was thin looking. Hunglu gazed into Lu's eyes. They were a deep green, like two dragon scales. Hunglu did not know whether to trust this man's words. But then again, did he have any choice?

Lu was almost thirty-five years old and had been trained to be a bodyguard by his father and grandfather from the age of six. The family had protected caravans for six generations and was considered the best escort service in southern China. Two years earlier, Lu's father had been killed escorting a caravan. His father had been in a backup position, disguised as a porter, when an ambush very similar to this one had occurred. The old man had been ready to kill an archer when he realized that the bandit was just a terrified boy. He had not been able to bring himself to kill someone so young.

"I give you your life today, boy. Go and do something good with it," he said as he let the boy go free.

The caravan regrouped and continued its journey. About a mile up the trail, the old man had been cleanly shot through the heart by the boy's arrow.

"Thank you, foolish old man," the boy had mocked from the trees. "Now I've done something good today!"

Since then, all bandits who attacked a caravan Lu escorted were killed without question.

From this story and many more he would hear in the coming days, Hunglu began to understand the role of good and evil in the world. The actions were often the same, only intentions made the difference. This was the beginning of his warrior training.

A few days after the attack, it was Lu who introduced Hunglu to the martial arts and its code of honor. He told Hunglu many stories about martial chivalry and personal battles. Lu told stories not to brag, but to teach techniques and tactics through his experience. Because of Hunglu's age and small stature, Lu thought it best to begin training him in the Tiger style of fighting.

The Tiger style was a system that developed muscular power and strength in the user. Every day before the caravan started out, Hunglu assumed deep, knee-bent postures while practicing various blocking and striking techniques with his hands formed into the shape of tiger claws. The exercises were foreign to him and his awkwardness showed. Already tired as the caravan set off, he then carried his porter loads for long hours. Then, after the day's work, Hunglu again practiced Tiger-form sets. He willingly accepted his lessons as they kept him too tired to think of his sad past and unpredictable future.

The form sets were most fascinating to Hunglu. He learned combinations of fighting techniques linked together to simulate a mock battle. Before the journey was over, Hunglu had become strong and muscular, but more importantly he had learned thirty Tiger-form sets.

Beyond martial arts, Lu also taught Hunglu to observe nature, to track men and animals, and to distinguish natural foliage from camouflage. These were invaluable skills that allowed men to see an ambush before it happened, thus removing the element of surprise. Hunglu learned quickly and was given a few defensive responsibilities should the caravan be attacked again. Lu explained that sometimes experience was the best teacher for fledgling warriors. All of Lu's training built Hunglu's confidence, and the responsibility began to make him feel more in control of his destiny.

Three days outside of Nanking, Lu warned Hunglu, "Be alert today, we are being followed."

Everyone was looking for the ambush, but Cheng saw it first. He noticed the misplaced grass around the base of a bush. He started singing a folk song as a warning to the rest of the caravan.

Hunglu, his nerves and senses heightened, observed the stillness of the birds just before the bandits charged.

Four swordsmen attacked quickly, coming from the trees, like flashes of silver light. A man with two crescent knives threatened the left side of the column. Another spearman appeared to the right side, where Hunglu was. Hunglu's assignment was to cover Lu should he move into action. Lu stayed motionless, acting like a frightened carrier.

Cheng single-handedly dispatched both swordsmen in the rear, while the left-rear guard, Lu's cousin, attacked the spearman. An arrow ripped through the cousin's leg. A second arrow flew over Hunglu's head from the left, just missing the cousin by inches. There were two archers this time—Hunglu had only expected and seen one archer. He now understood why Lu had not committed to an attack. Hunglu felt the weight of his inexperience and insecurity suddenly filled his mind. He was terrified of what would happen next.

Cheng attracted the archers' attention next as he ran between the two horses in the rear and removed a bow from his pack. Two arrows fired by both archers simultaneously struck the horse Cheng was behind. Before the horse even hit the ground, the archer on the right was dead from one of Cheng's arrows.

By this time the right front guard had killed his attacker and was charging into the woods, where the second archer was. The other front guard was still engaged with his bandit. Lu didn't move, but neither did the bandit with the crescent knives.

Two horsemen who were swirling long-handled Kwando swords charged from the woods, attacking Cheng and the right front guard. Cheng's second arrow found its mark, killing the left archer. By diving behind a tree, only barely was Cheng able to avoid the Kwando attack.

Finally, the bandit with the crescent knives moved. It was a fatal error. He went after Cheng, who appeared to be busy fending off another mounted attack.

Lu quickly grabbed Cheng's sword from behind the dead horse and tossed it to him. Lu's sudden motions re-attracted the crescent-knife bandit, who now realized that the man who seemed to be a frightened porter was actually a part of the caravan's defense. With knives flashing, he turned to attack. Removing the twin daggers from his waistband, Lu parried the slashing combinations. The bandit was well trained and kept Lu busy.

While Lu's back was turned, the spearman rushed forward. Almost without thinking, Hunglu grabbed the spear as the thief charged past. Using his training, Hunglu was able to redirect the shaft into the ground, and as the spearman stumbled Hunglu caught him in the throat with his elbow, dropping the man to his knees. Channeling all his fear, rage, and strength, Hunglu struck the spearman on the side of his head with a right tiger paw. His palm crushed into the thief's head, fatally fracturing the man's skull. The surprisingly soft feeling of his hand going into another man's head frightened Hunglu and for a moment he felt as if he had committed the worst mistake in his life. At the same time, Hunglu was fascinated by the ease of his actions; the thick skull barely resisted the force of his Tiger technique. He had felt the bones in the man's head shatter, a feeling that still reverberated in his arm.

Lu managed to cut the left wrist of his attacker and was about to launch a death combination when the front horseman attacked with his Kwando. Hunglu grabbed the spear from his fallen attacker and thrust it into the horseman's ribs. At the same moment, Lu's dagger pierced the crescent-knife bandit's heart.

The momentum of the charging horseman forced Hunglu into the ground and pulled the spear from his hands. He had been holding the spear so tight that his shoulder was dislocated before he could let go. Breathless and confused, Hunglu lay in the dirt, writhing in pain. He wondered now if he would die like the victim he just dispatched.

The fight nearly complete, Cheng grabbed a fallen tree limb and threw it at the face of his attacker's horse. The flying limb frightened the horse, causing it to rear up and throw the surprised rider. When the rider struck the ground, Cheng's sword was there to meet him.

Lu ran over to Hunglu and cradled him in his arms. He quickly searched Hunglu for injuries and discovered the dislocated shoulder. Taking the twisted arm in his hands, Lu cautioned, "Don't move,

Hunglu, this will hurt!" Then he snapped the joint back into place. Hunglu's strong, newly developed muscles spasmed with incredible pain. He was barely able to suppress a scream. Listening to the shouts of victory around him, Hunglu lapsed into unconsciousness. A deep, black void surrounded him, but there was a distant flicker of light . . .

In his private courtyard next to the monastery, Hunglu's mind returned from the past as he finished his Tai Chi form. He felt re-invigorated. He looked at the sleeping parrot. The valley was peaceful. It seemed to Hunglu that an eternity had passed since that first battle.

Looking back, the journey to his uncle's was a way of armoring his heart against his past. His father had tossed Hunglu out of the family, and that action caused the boy to lose his innocence on the road. It was the beginning of many horrors he would both see *and* do to others in his lifetime.

For many years Hunglu took pride in the fighting prowess he displayed on the day of the ambush. He had, with very little training and experience, successfully defeated experienced bandits in battle. Now, from a perspective provided by maturity, he realized he had only been lucky. There were five other men there who could have helped and who didn't fight. In fact, Cheng and Lu alone could have handled the situation. But Hunglu joined the battle with little hesitation. What were his true motives, he wondered. It could have been for survival, but still five other men didn't fight and *they* survived. The trader, a seasoned soldier who was armed and mounted, had just sat and watched. Yet was the trader ever in any danger? Hunglu tried to remember.

Perhaps it was because fighting was the right thing to do that Hunglu joined the battle. That sounded true for a moment, but it wasn't. The truth, Hunglu finally decided, was that he had wanted honor. He wanted it like a possession to carry and show others who might question his purpose on earth.

His father thought he was worthless. So Hunglu had solicited these powerful men to train him. Hunglu fought to prove his power, and in so doing, he would prove his value. But to what end? Hunglu's father never knew of this courage, this newfound prowess. Hunglu could demonstrate his usefulness to Lu and Cheng, but he could not replace a pear with a carrot—Lu and Cheng were not his father.

Hunglu began to understand what the Butterfly Immortal had meant in their last meeting: *Avoidance of pain is our motivation to action.* Perhaps this was why Hunglu was so eager to accept that early violence. In it he found the surrogate bonds for his lost family. Neither Lu nor Cheng, two men dear to Hunglu, could ever replace his real family, though. It was foolish to think so. There were no bonds greater than those of blood relations. At best, he had achieved only camaraderie. He was still alone in the world.

Hunglu sat back beneath a tree and began to breathe, clearing his mind and focusing upon the question, "What do I *need* to know right now?"

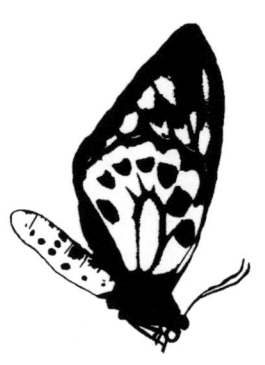

THE WAX HEART

He found himself in the fields outside his childhood home. There was a young man working the fields and a pretty woman nursing a baby. An older child, a little boy of about three, was running up and down the crop rows.

Hunglu tried to determine where he was in time. With only his intuition to process his surroundings, he decided he was in the present time and the events he was seeing were occurring at that very moment.

For a long time Hunglu watched the young couple working the farm, wondering who they were. He wandered over to the house. A dog saw him approach and stood up and growled.

"I mean your family no harm," Hunglu said in a spirit voice.

The dog eyed him cautiously, then recognizing Hunglu's innate goodness, the animal wagged its tail.

Hunglu entered the house through a wall. He saw a man about ten years older than he, sitting with a cup of tea. A scan of the man's body revealed that he was very sick with a weak heart that prevented him from doing anything but the simplest of activities. Hunglu tried to see the life force within the body and recognized the energy as his oldest stepbrother. This definitely was his old home.

But who was the man in the field? Hunglu concentrated so hard on the man's face that he did not even feel his spirit body transported to the field. But then Hunglu was in front of the man, looking into his eyes. Yes, without a doubt, those were his *father's* eyes in the man.

Hunglu was moved by this realization. He always thought he would resent and even hate his half-brother, the product of his father and a hateful woman. Hunglu hovered in his ethereal state, waiting for violent emotions to rise up in him. Instead, an unexpected and wonderful truth came forward: he wanted to love his brother. The only violence Hunglu felt was the tremendous force from which the love poured from him. He reached out to the brother, who sensed nothing as Hunglu's arms passed through the farmer's body.

Shaken, Hunglu moved quickly backward and was stopped by another presence.

"Hello my son."

Hunglu turned to face the spirit of his mother.

She smiled warmly. "You need to see some things to have a better understanding of your life."

Hunglu's mother took him into the kitchen of their old house. There, Hunglu saw his father as he last left him, over twenty years before. Hungling was still a young man. His black hair was clipped close to his scalp, his shoulders broad and strong. Clearly, the moment was far in the past.

Hungling was arguing with Sunyin—an argument Hunglu's father was losing. Hungling had tears in his eyes as Sunyin passionately told him that she could not live with Hunglu anymore: "He does nothing. He is too weak to work in the fields!" she complained. "His mind wanders all the time, and he just sits there in his own world. I'm sorry, but his hard birth must have damaged his head. He talks crazy, and sees things that aren't there, Hungling."

"That is his gift," Hungling said in defense.

"It is his sickness! Do you want this crazy boy to lose all you have worked for?" Sunyin shot back. "His uncle is crazy too! They will make a fine pair together."

Hunglu's childhood rage was bubbling over. He wished he could reach into the vision and snap Sunyin's neck.

"What hurts you, Hunglu?" his mother asked.

"I am angry that she betrayed me," he seethed. "And he . . . *he* is weak."

"You are hurt. Your anger comes from your pain," Hunglu's mother said gently. "But why do you hurt so?"

"No one understood me or accepted me," Hunglu sighed.

"Your father did."

"How so? He tossed me out of my home for that woman."

"He saved you." Hunglu's mother explained softly.

She directed him to look to the left. Hunglu gazed in the direction his mother was pointing. He knew this place. It was the gallery where he battled the dragon. Now, though, he was a spectator watching his own great violent acts. His skills were mesmerizing, but his fury frightening.

The audience was consumed by the passion of the battle. They did not hear or see Hunglu's reluctance. As they watched him climb to the dragon's head and raise his blade, they screamed, "Kill! Kill! Kill!" Only when the sword struck home did the spectators roar their approval of him. Hunglu could feel the frenzy of the audience, but they were totally unaware of the suffering endured by both the dragon and its killer. The agony of murdering the crippled, defenseless dragon returned full force.

"Why can't they see what's happening?" He turned to meet his mother's eyes, pleading for an answer.

The scene faded as Hunglu's mother spoke. "People see only what they believe to be true. And their beliefs are created by their fears. For many months, your father believed you to be dead on your journey to Nanking. For many months he too felt as if he were dead. He did not want to sacrifice you, it was not he who wanted you gone."

She showed Hunglu a sequence of images. He watched as his father received a letter from Hunglu's uncle in Nanking. Hungling trembled with relief as he read that Hunglu had arrived safely. Then Hungling folded the letter as small as he could and melted red sealing wax over the paper, building layer upon layer, until it was preserved in a hard shell. It looked like a tiny heart.

Hunglu watched each day of his father's life flashing by. And each day his father removed the wax-covered letter from his belt pouch and prayed for Hunglu's safety and welfare. The images slowed down as Hungling fell ill. Soon he began the agonizing process of dying. Hunglu watched his father's last breath on earth. Wasted and weakened, Hungling gripped the wax-covered letter in his hand and held it in the air, as if an offering to the gods. When Sunyin entered the room she knew that he was gone. She raced to the bed and tore at Hungling's fist. But in death Hungling was too strong, and Sunyin could not pry the secret letter from his lifeless body.

Now Hunglu understood. His father *had* wanted him. The knowledge simultaneously filled him with happiness and sadness. He wished that he could find his father and apologize. Perhaps his mother could help, but when Hunglu looked back for her, she was gone.

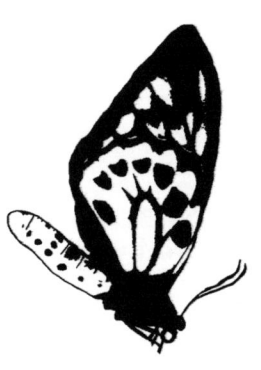

WU CHIENHUO

He had discovered that his father truly loved and accepted him. Deep within his heart, Hunglu had always known this to be true, but the pain of abandonment masked this knowledge all his life. It was he who created the belief that his father didn't accept him, and he created that belief out of fear—fear that the person he loved and trusted could leave him, betray him.

Hunglu's mother had loved and nurtured him, and then she died. His father had loved him, then deserted him for another family. These painful experiences caused Hunglu to search for ways to prevent further pain in his life. He allowed himself to become numb to his past. But his training as a monk made Hunglu acknowledge that his experience did, in fact, exist—love survived distance and death. The workings of the Tao required each person to be courageous, to have the strength to do the right action no matter what pain might be perceived or endured. Yet, he was unable to completely embrace this idea until he met his master. Now he saw more clearly than he ever thought possible.

Hunglu wanted to thank the Butterfly Immortal for this gift of sight. In the last two days, he had experienced more emotions than he had in the past twenty years. It was painful reviewing these pivotal memories, but at the same time he was feeling more alive than ever before. He had a great desire to seek out the Butterfly Immortal and tell the master that he had learned the lesson well. Hunglu did not know that the lessons had only just begun.

For the moment, Hunglu reveled in the idea that his father was courageous—in life *and* death. Hungling had to accept the pain of loss too. If not for Hungling's courage, Hunglu would have been a farmer, never having the advantages, education, or experiences that made him what he was. Without his father, Hunglu knew he would never have done the things he held most dear. No, it was not his destiny to be a farmer.

Hunglu continued to ponder all he would have missed if he had been a farmer. In the end, Hunglu concluded that his greatest loss would have been not meeting Wu Chienhuo.

Hunglu's uncle was excited to receive news that his nephew was coming to live with him. Wu Chienhuo fathered four daughters and no sons, so the prospect of having an heir pleased him, especially the son of his sister, Little Fawn.

Little Fawn was ten years younger than he and the eighth child in the family. Chienhuo saw a sensitive and beautiful spirit in his sister. Throughout her short life, he was committed to protecting that spirit. He helped to raise her, and educated her beyond the normal limits imposed on her gender. They were best friends. In choosing to take in Hunglu, he reasoned that the son of his sister would also possess creativity and intelligence—skills that Chienhuo could nurture and use.

Chienhuo encouraged Little Fawn's marriage to Hungling. He respected Hungling and admired his ambition and his successes. He knew Hungling would take care of his sister and, above all, nurture her tender-loving spirit. So shortly after Little Fawn married, Chienhuo moved out of the village to pursue greater opportunities in Nanking.

Wu Chienhuo was the second son in the family and had learned the trade of his father, a brickmaker and stone worker. He loved to build and especially craved the challenge of erecting complex structures and bridges.

There were many difficult building projects in the southern capital, and Chienhuo rose to the opportunity. His creative designs and knowledge of materials allowed him to construct buildings others couldn't even imagine. Among peasants and lords alike, he became known as the Builder of Dreams.

Within twenty years, Wu Chienhuo established a formidable reputation, raised a small family, and amassed a considerable amount of political power. A result of his talent and connections was that he received special imperial projects.

Chienhuo was also known for his personal discipline and an uncanny ability to gather and direct talented individuals. People *wanted* to work for him because he would bring out their best and reward them for it. He was loved by his workers and became a legend among the peasant class because of his rags-to-riches success.

Determined to give Hunglu the education, training, and advantages of an adopted son, Chienhuo prepared for the boy's arrival.

When Hunglu arrived in Nanking, he was still nursing his bruised shoulder with an inflated ego—he believed he had become a man along the journey, a self-sufficient being. There was little in life that could surprise him. But as Hunglu rode through the gate onto his uncle's property, his ego started melting.

"Are you sure this is the right place?" he asked the escort beside him. "This looks like an imperial palace."

Chienhuo's home was in fact a miniature version of the Southern Palace, complete with gardens and peacocks.

"This all belongs to your uncle," the escort said. "You are very fortunate."

Hunglu turned to Lu, who was also accompanying him in this last leg of their journey. "Did you know my uncle was so wealthy?"

"Who do you think paid for us?" Lu said, smiling.

Over the many months of his journey to Nanking, Hunglu had wondered how a small trader with so few goods could afford such seasoned, high-quality guards.

"You were our most prized merchandise," Lu said. "But you gave us quite a scare the other day."

Chienhuo greeted Hunglu and Lu in the main hall. He was a powerfully muscled forty-six-year-old man who looked more like a stonecutter than the royalty Hunglu expected after seeing the estate. Chienhuo still spent many hours working with his men; it was his disposition to be a part of the action, to never forget his beginnings.

Chienhuo ran over to his nephew and lifted him into his arms with a ferocious hug. This both surprised and embarrassed Hunglu in front of his comrades. At the same time, his body melted into the loving embrace. Not since his mother had anyone been so glad to see him. Hunglu knew in an instant that he would like his uncle.

A formal banquet was prepared in Hunglu's honor. It was like nothing he had ever seen. Roasted peacocks glazed with honey and decorated with herbs filled the tables. Flasks of ruby-colored wine endlessly drained into finely cut goblets glittering in candlelight.

Guests arrived in magnificent garbs. There was music and dancing, and entertainers roaming about the enormous grand hall. Hunglu had never seen such finery and splendor. He never imagined that *his* family would be so wealthy, or for that matter what wealth really was. After dinner, Chienhuo made Hunglu stand in front of the nearly fifty guests from the finer social ranks in Nanking. Timidly, Hunglu rose, though he could not bring himself to look directly into the faces of those around him.

"Men and women of Nanking—my friends—I am pleased to introduce you to my nephew, Hunglu." Turning to Hunglu, Chienhuo said, "Welcome to our family!"

The guests stood up, applauding and beaming at the small, shy boy before them.

Hunglu looked up and smiled winningly—his natural timidity worked to his advantage, endearing him to others. He had no idea of the implications of Chienhuo's introduction; Hunglu was just pleased to have a family again. His future and position within the elite of Nanking had just been assured, but all he knew was that he was finally wanted.

The next three years were spent in intensive training to develop Hunglu's mind. Chienhuo hired the best tutors to teach Hunglu mathematics, classics, and engineering. He was taken to construction sites three days a week to get his hands dirty and learn the basic rules of his new trade.

On Hunglu's eighteenth birthday, Chienhuo sent his nephew to work on a large imperial project in a western province. The project was the construction of a small city. Hunglu was assigned to learn and work every job, from the lowest position to supervisor.

Hunglu loved learning the trades. It was work that had meaning and that displayed measurable results for his toils. His mind found focus and direction, occulting all thoughts and pains from his past. He made walls, bridges, and gardens with his own hands, creating lasting objects where there had been nothing. Hunglu found it very satisfying to look at his day's work and see it slowly accumulate into magnificent settings. He often spent his quiet hours in contemplation among his creations, trying to understand the meaning of things and especially the actions of people. More and more he was feeling a great compulsion to grasp the fundamentals of human nature. It was his belief that if he could understand the likes and desires of people he could design better and more appealing structures. But most of all he just liked people and living a simple life.

The men with whom Hunglu worked were authentic, not like the men of Nanking who were filled with inflated language, obscure concepts, and vague ideas about their spirituality. The workers, spoke about what they believed in with tremendous passion, and they only believed what they saw. There was a genuineness about them that he admired. He felt comfortable in their midst and enjoyed their simple but elegant talk. Hunglu tried to fit in with these men and their beliefs. Yet at the same time, the hard work within these beautiful, natural surroundings was stimulating Hunglu's visions and thirst for spiritual adventures. Clairvoyant visions often occurred in his dreams, foretelling dangers on the job. Hunglu used this knowledge to quietly intervene to prevent serious accidents. He was cautious. He didn't want to be mistrusted or ridiculed by his co-workers. Hunglu believed these practical men would never be able to understand the visions or him, so he moved silently behind the scenes.

His opinion of the men's character changed one day when Hunglu overheard a big bull of a worker named Ox yell up to a man on the scaffolding, "Yang, get down from there! Last night, I dreamed you fell from that spot."

Yang immediately got off the scaffolding. The men inspected the apparatus and discovered that some of the ropes holding it were rotted and weak. Without any discussion or ceremony, the ropes were quickly replaced and work went on as normal. Hunglu was amazed by the lack of reaction to this profound warning. He talked to one of the supervisors about it.

"These warnings happen all the time, Hunglu," the supervisor said nonchalantly. "Every man has dreams and silly ideas about doing things better. That is the way things are. It's foolish to ask questions; we just respect and follow our hearts."

Hunglu heard many exciting stories after this event. Although the men wholeheartedly accepted their unexplained visions, they were quick to characterize the spiritualists as fools. The workers were pragmatic men who believed in things that produced results and could be *seen* and *used*. This included visions that had both practical and personal value. They believed in personal miracles, not in theories, philosophies, or men who thought they were smart enough to know the unknowable.

Hunglu's teachers in Nanking were different. They eagerly believed in ancient theories and philosophies. They often debated for hours over nuances of the same thought, dazzling themselves with their own rhetorical acrobatics and understanding of how the universe worked. These men always demanded facts and proof to support the opinions of others. Nothing was immediately acceptable, and the search for answers to all questions was endless.

Among the common workers, Hunglu observed that facts and proof really didn't matter at all. The men of Nanking would only believe what they wanted to believe. If the evidence was against them, the men would then dispute the validity of the facts. And if that was unsuccessful, they would attack the credibility of the man with the facts. Anything that supported their beliefs was true and wise; anything that did not was false and its followers fools. At eighteen, Hunglu was excited about this rebellious attitude. He had met a lot of fools in his three years in Nanking. Now he was with wise men who knew their worth.

However, as Hunglu progressed upward in the trades he again found fools, men who tried to emulate the attitudes of the scholars but lacked the intelligence to even create a half-way believable persona. It seemed that the more successful one was, the more he was prone to straying farther from what was simple and obvious to everyone. Hunglu thought it must be a horror to live as some of these men with high status. Did they even know how ignorant they appeared to the rest of the world? He resolved never to delve too deeply into spiritual matters. To accept or deny experiences based on his initial instinct seemed far more appropriate to the young man. To overanalyze anything was nothing more than an exercise in futility.

After six years of arduous work, Hunglu had experienced and learned the basic skills of every trade within the new city. He had earned and was given supervisory status and started designing his own buildings. Hunglu had won the respect of everyone on his projects for his ability to learn, understand, and apply what he had been taught. But an old stonecutter summed it up best for Hunglu: "I've been working for your uncle for twenty years. You are wise like him because you respect and listen to people. As long as you continue to listen to what others tell you, you will be successful."

Chienhuo brought Hunglu back to Nanking when he was twenty-four. To complete his training, Hunglu needed to learn large-scale management of business. The boy who left Nanking was now a strong, practical man with many building and design skills. During Hunglu's absence, the emperor had appointed Chienhuo as a minister of building. With his increased political duties and growing list of building projects, Chienhuo needed access to Hunglu's skills. It was also important to teach Hunglu political and social skills that would prepare him to be an heir and carry on the Wu Chienhuo prosperity.

Under his uncle's tutelage, Hunglu soon learned to manipulate the influential persons of Nanking. This ability surprised Hunglu. Within himself he recognized a great power. It was dizzyingly easy to make people do what he wanted them to do. Part of his skill was to appear charmingly shy, like he had when he first arrived in Nanking. Only now it was an act. His shyness made others feel as if they were in control of the situation. Meanwhile, Hunglu goaded them into seeing his point of view while never quite being aggressive. It was his peculiar ability to make people feel much better about being in the wrong than they had felt being in the right. It was a dangerous power for a young man to have, but Hunglu maintained it responsibly. He did not like the fact that he had to manipulate others to do what was wise and right.

Chienhuo complimented Hunglu on his political skills so profusely that Hunglu didn't have the heart to confess his distaste for making deals. Hunglu sometimes wondered if anyone suspected he held a slight contempt for business, and almost imperceptibly, he began to recede from his manufactured persona. Uncomfortable questions entered his mind, such as was this all there was to master in the world?

Noticing his nephew's waning enthusiasm, Chienhuo hoped Hunglu would eventually find a wife. A wife could quell his doubts and re-ignite Hunglu's spirit of competition. A good wife would be there to listen to her husband at night, to share his worries and discomforts so he did not have to bear his burdens alone. The two of them would team against the world when necessary and a woman of class and cunning could help a man like Hunglu to discover unlimited power and happiness. Sometimes a man needed a woman to remind him of what was important. It appeared that Hunglu had a promising future ahead of him, and Chienhuo thought that finding a wife for his nephew would be no problem.

But Hunglu did not express interest in the women that Chienhuo brought to the house. Instead, Hunglu's mind was focused on learning this new business environment. His work now involved the mind, not the hands. He was occupied every moment with planning and organizing projects around the region. In maintaining his uncle's empire, Hunglu had no time for women. More often than not, he was simply too exhausted to even long for one. After a while, Chienhuo stopped bringing women into Hunglu's life. His nephew barely seemed to notice, which saddened the old man. He wanted his nephew to be happy; if not with the companionship of a woman, perhaps he could offer Hunglu more power. He did not suspect that Hunglu would desire anything other than a woman or power—what else was there?

Chienhuo became more involved in political affairs, leaving most of the management and design responsibilities to Hunglu. Hunglu's existence, in turn, was consumed with details and tasks from waking to sleep. He no longer worked surrounded by beautiful scenery, and there were no more peaceful visions, no more straightforward men. Everyone he met now had an agenda and a secret.

The burden of dealing with insincere people took its toll. First he became disconnected from nature—he rarely was aware of the time of day or the weather outside. Then he lost touch with his body. His once strong and supple physique had become stiff, slow, and flabby. Then his passions failed. It seemed he was just a fat husk of a person with no visions for the future and no passion to do anything. He slogged forward through a swamp of duties and responsibilities. With increased responsibility, he had less opportunity to work with design and absolutely no opportunity to work with the tradesmen. The two things he most loved about his career were now unavailable to him. He had become an imperial administrator; he was no longer a living man.

When life seemed its worst, a war erupted, and Hunglu snapped out of his haze.

Warlords in the eastern provinces had formed an alliance and were waging a campaign of rebellion against the southern capital. It was their objective to control the southern provinces, thus governing access to trade with all of southeast Asia. This plan, if successful, would strangle the empire and end the existing dynasty. The emperor sent his two most trusted warlord allies to engage the enemy and conquer them.

It was a time when the price of a warlord's loyalty was political favors, not honor. These men could easily turn for greater rewards if the tide of battle shifted against them. It was the emperor's only hope that an imperial army could be developed before Nanking was lost. Conscription was enacted in the southern provinces to raise an army for the empire.

Though immune to the draft, Hunglu's loyalty to the emperor, his belief in martial chivalry, and an incredible need to escape his current life pushed him to volunteer for service. When he heard the news, Chienhuo was outraged at the irresponsible and dangerous act.

"I will not lose my son to greed and false honor!" Chienhuo shouted.

"Uncle, I will be fighting to preserve our life and our emperor," Hunglu argued calmly. He began to sort through weapons he accumulated throughout the years. Most of them were ceremonial gifts: honorary swords, ornate daggers, brass shields, and the like. In times of war, the tools of violence were valuable only for their destructive power.

"I forbid you to go!" his uncle raged.

"We have too much to lose," Hunglu said. "Look around you, Uncle. Do you possibly think we will survive should Nanking and the emperor fall?"

This was a telling point. Chienhuo had dined with the emperor many times and realized his head would not stay long upon his shoulders if the army failed to defend Nanking. But still, Chienhuo was not prepared to lose his adopted son.

"Hunglu, there are enough men to fight this war, *you* do not have to go," he pleaded.

"Uncle, just as we have worked side by side with our men, we owe it to them to be with them in battle," Hunglu countered. "All of our principles, all of our respect, would be sacrificed, if we did not do our part. It is you who taught me this."

Both sadness and pride appeared on the face of Chienhuo. "You have grown into a wise man, and I have become too old and foolish to see the truth. I know you are very unhappy with your life right now, and I have refused to see your unhappiness. I mistakenly have forced my dreams upon your destiny."

"Parents are often guilty of this injustice," Hunglu callously reflected. He immediately regretted what he said and turned to his uncle. "I am sorry. You have given me so much. Now give me your blessing and pray for my safe and speedy return."

Chienhuo's eyes watered, unable to contain the tears of his loss.

Hunglu was shocked by Chienhuo's full expression of emotions—it nearly made him begin to put his weapons away.

Most men repressed these emotions so as not to reveal a weakness; this is what Hunglu believed his father had done when he sent Hunglu to Wu Chienhuo. But unlike Hungling, Hunglu knew Chienhuo had no weaknesses to hide. He moved forward and embraced Chienhuo, the man who had given him more than he could have ever imagined.

GRANDMASTER

Hunglu spent the afternoon showing the parrot how to find food in its natural surroundings. The parrot had grown quickly. Its widening breast was a vibrant blue, like the color of royal garbs. The parrot was also growing in confidence, swooping about the cabin like an azure streak of light. Sometimes it would dive from the rafters onto Hunglu's shoulders, beating its powerful wings and sending cool waves of air down his back.

Although the bird looked like an adult, it was still too young to forage and feed itself, so it was necessary to take the parrot on food-discovery trips and teach it what to look for. Finding food, above all else, was the single most important skill the bird would have to learn.

Walking through the woods with the bird fluttering from tree branch to tree branch, Hunglu reminisced about his uncle. Chienhuo had given him everything, but the most important gift he gave was love. Hunglu had never felt so completely loved and accepted since leaving his uncle. He had, in fact, been so occupied trying to avoid love that he hadn't realized how loved he had been in life. Chienhuo demonstrated the power of truth that the Butterfly Immortal had alluded to. His complete emotional expression made Chienhuo creditable to those who knew him, allowing him to release negative feelings directly, and putting him in the powerful position of always speaking from the truth. Chienhuo's men liked working for him, not because of his wealth and position, but because he was authentic and sincerely cared for them. Hunglu's uncle was truly a master of the art of truth, happily and effortlessly sailing through his incredible life by living a doctrine of love and acceptance that transcended social boundaries. He did not have to create artificial personas to accomplish his goals; Chienhuo was true to himself, and therein lay his power.

When a person became adept at hiding feelings, Hunglu realized, he only succeeded in hiding the truth about himself. Hidden feelings created beliefs and behaviors that did not necessarily support life's purpose; however, they did prevent a person from touching upon unpleasant feelings. That is what made them so appealing, but also so dangerous. A person could waste an entire lifetime running away from feelings and truth. Hunglu knew that this was one of his errors.

Through Chienhuo's influence, Hunglu had learned how people lived and thought at all levels of society. He had worked with imperial ministers and indentured slaves and found them to be not so different. Once one subtracted the basic need for food and shelter, Hunglu observed, all the other issues in life were the same. Each person was indeed dedicated to their emotions and fears. Whether rich, noble, or poor, each person was still just human. After reflecting upon all his interactions with the high-placed men of Nanking, Hunglu realized how obvious that truth was. They all seemed to have a tension, as if they were hiding something. Now he recognized that what they were hiding was their truth, their emotions. And Hunglu, overwhelmed by the tasks he had taken on, had started to act in the same manner. If it had not been for the war, he knew he would have lost himself completely.

After the parrot had found sufficient sustenance for the day, Hunglu returned to the main complex to gather some grain for himself and talk to the Grandmaster.

The monastery was a U-shaped arrangement of sand-colored buildings. In the center was the main temple, behind which was the kitchen. A monk's diet consisted of simple foods, mostly porridges and cakes made from grains and vegetables. One of Hunglu's community tasks was to cultivate the gardens that supplied the vegetables for the brothers. Gardening, like building, connected him to the earth and made him feel productive. Sometimes he would work for hours, sifting the dirt until it was dark and silky. He planted seeds with careful attention to where they lay in relation to the sun and the shadows of the temple. Then he crept among the plants, the fierce sun beating down on his scarred back, inspecting them for fungus or parasites. During the growing season, he was at one with the land and could again see the results of his efforts. It was a peaceful, pristine time for him.

The parrot followed Hunglu into the lush gardens. It fluttered down on a tomato plant and tore the rind with its yellow beak, but Hunglu gave the bird a stern look. "That is not for you, little one. That is for my *other* brothers."

The parrot lifted off and together they entered the kitchen. A wizened man named Old Cook was busy preparing a mountainous salad. His small, pale body was contrary to the classic image of a well-fed chef. But Old Cook had always been contrary to most of what was expected of him. He did not even seem to care too much about the meals he made and often complained about the lack of good ingredients. But the monks knew that this was a façade manufactured to keep them away from the kitchen and out of Old Cook's way.

"Yes, yes," Old Cook often grumbled to himself over his raw ingredients. "My brothers will get what they get. It is not my job to feed them like kings."

But Old Cook always *did* feed the men like kings. What looked like a simple salad actually contained a myriad of flavors, each blending in magical wonderment with the next, the taste and texture perfectly balanced with the rest of the meal. He was loved by the brothers as much for culinary creations as his gruff humor.

"Oh, I see you bring me meat for dinner, Flying Spirit!" barked Old Cook when he saw Hunglu enter the kitchen.

Hunglu was confused by the statement at first. Then the parrot squawked and violently beat his wings at the old man.

"Yes, I hear you bird," Old Cook said. "If you don't leave my kitchen, you will be in my soup."

"You've offended him, Old Cook," Hunglu said, smiling.

Old Cook grabbed a cleaver and feigning fear shouted, "Last warning: you get that vicious bird out of my kitchen!"

The mock threats of the cook made Hunglu roar with laughter until his sides hurt. His reaction triggered a mass attack of giggles by others in the kitchen.

Old Cook, a natural comic always looking for an audience, was tickled with himself. Hunglu had always proved difficult to make laugh—he was always so thoughtful or just plain absent from what was going on. To catch him like this really pleased Old Cook.

"Okay, I'll let your bird live for today, Hunglu," he said.

The Grandmaster, who had been walking by the kitchen, was attracted by the laughter and entered. He saw Hunglu holding his stomach, struggling to catch his breath, and laughing silently. The Grandmaster could not contain his own laughter.

The parrot, assuming the commotion was an important call of its flock, enthusiastically joined in with its own screeching version of laughter. Just when everyone was getting control of themselves, the parrot's spontaneously poor imitation of Hunglu's laugh set them all off again.

This is good, thought the Grandmaster. He always had a great desire to see Hunglu at ease with his brothers.

After recovering his breath, Hunglu gathered a ration of grain and rice, teasing Old Cook. "Give me more rice, master, or I'll set my bird on you!"

Then with his rations in hand and bird upon his shoulder, Hunglu walked out with the Grandmaster through the gardens.

"It is so good to see you laugh, Hunglu," the Grandmaster commented. "It tells me that you are doing well with your lessons."

"I'm not doing any work at all," Hunglu confessed. "I'm just daydreaming about my past."

"*Ahhhh.* If that is what the Butterfly Immortal instructed you to do, you must do it."

"Grandmaster, what do you mean by saying I'm doing well with my lessons?"

"Flying Spirit," the Grandmaster began, "you spend too much time with your mind outside of your body, not in spiritual travel, but avoiding life. You have become lost in your thoughts and lack real interaction with others. The only time you are present in the moment is when you practice your martial arts or work in the garden. When you were laughing in there, Hunglu, you were in the present— physically, mentally, and spiritually. Didn't it *feel* more real to you?"

Of course the Grandmaster was correct: Hunglu did feel more real, more alive. It was almost like his mental haze was lifted, a haze that painfully and frustratingly separated him from others.

"Yes, it was more real," Hunglu agreed, "but I don't understand why."

The Grandmaster explained: "The mind provides direction for the body and spirit within the physical life. Both the body and the spirit will follow the focus of the mind, and where the spirit goes, its vital energy will follow. A mind that is always focused outside the body will direct the spirit outside the body. A mind that is unfocused causes disruption of body and spirit. An orderly mind focused within the body provides balance of mind, body, and spirit, resulting in optimum health. So how we *think* has a great effect on our life." The Grandmaster paused. "Similarly, a mind only focused on the future carries the vital energy of the spirit forward into the future. This can be good if the energy is channeled to create a positive future. But it is bad if the energy is wasted on idle dreaming. In either case energy leaves the body, which can drain it, leaving it vulnerable to illness and incapable of functioning effectively in the present."

"What about focusing on the past," Hunglu asked.

"The same is true, except the past cannot be changed. Unless self-knowledge is gained, focusing on the past is a foolish waste of energy."

Hunglu began to worry. "So my lack of attention is hurting my body?"

"Not permanently," answered the Grandmaster. "You re-balance your body with your Chi Kung exercises. But you, Hunglu, have been intentionally escaping from your life."

"If I have, I don't know why," Hunglu said.

"That is what you are going to find out through your life review," the Grandmaster reminded him. "You cannot know where you are going until you know where you have been. To go on a journey you must know where you are and how you have gotten there. By reviewing your life you can discover what fears have created your beliefs and motivations. Once you discover these veils, only then can you find your soul's personality and its unique purpose."

"*Veils?*" mumbled Hunglu.

"Veils are used to prevent someone from having a clear image of what's underneath. In martial arts, you practice a technique over and over until it becomes an instinct. When you are attacked, the defensive technique you learned happens without conscious intervention." The Grandmaster moved his hands in an example of a mock martial application to emphasize his point. "You are trained by your parents and village in how to behave and react in life. These trained responses, like fighting techniques, ensure your safety within your village. They allow you to blend into your village and family like a bird blends into a flock. You must know the proper calls to be accepted by the flock. But they cover, or veil, your soul's responses. Of course some of the training is in harmony with the soul and its purpose. But it is from your soul that your truth comes, and if the veil over the soul is too dense you can *never* see your true self."

Hunglu stopped and looked at the Grandmaster. "Yet, if I help my soul achieve its purpose, won't I die sooner?"

"Not so!" the Grandmaster laughed. "Not so! You will receive more training on the soul later. Now you must concentrate on your life review to remove the veils and discover who you are at your soul level. The review will reveal your underlying nature and allow you to discover your true purpose."

"I thought I already discovered my purpose," Hunglu stammered. "I've chosen the life of a monk and teacher."

"*Who* chose?" the Grandmaster demanded.

"I chose," Hunglu said, confused.

"And who is *I*? Flying Spirit, purpose is not a choice. It strikes you and compels you to do its bidding, with or without your conscious choice," the Grandmaster lectured. "Continue reviewing your life; it is the most important spiritual exercise you will ever do. And keep that vicious bird away from Old Cook!" With that the Grandmaster smiled and walked away.

The weight of the Grandmaster's last words bore heavily upon Hunglu. He had not considered in seven years that he was not fulfilling his purpose. This realization was very disconcerting. What possible options were left to him? What purpose was higher than spiritual service as a monk? Hunglu thought the Grandmaster must have meant that *truth* was more important than *choice*. He specifically said that purpose compelled humans to do its bidding. Suddenly Hunglu realized that this was what happened to him.

The young monk decided to walk around the western side of the mountain to catch the sunset and to recall the events that brought him to this monastery.

GENERAL KWAN

General Kwan Shandao was sent by the emperor to raise an army in Nanking and launch an attack on the eastern warlords. His other primary duty was to keep the emperor's allies in check. General Kwan was the direct descendant of the great General Kwan Tzu, inventor of the Kwando and undefeated master of military tactics. But General Kwan believed that he was not just a descendant of the great general, but actually Kwan Tzu's reincarnation. Watching him, it was hard to believe he wasn't.

Kwan, like his ancestor, was a master of tactics and very creative in the course of battle. He mastered the ancestral weapon of his family, the Kwando, a wide-bladed twenty-five-inch sword mounted on the end of a five-foot steel or wooden pole. It was primarily used from horseback and could be utilized against foot solders. However, the Kwando was equally effective against mounted warriors: one swing could easily chop off a horse's leg.

General Kwan's Kwando was particularly heavy, being made from the finest steel available, yet he wielded it faster than most men could use a small sword. An imperial historian once watched General Kwan single-handedly kill over one hundred men in a battle that lasted two hours. Since then, he had earned the name Blood Demon, as the ground he tread was always left saturated with blood. A mass of severed limbs and heads infallibly indicated his presence on the battlefield. Plain and simple General Kwan was a killing machine.

Now the general stood on a platform, wearing brightly colored but scarred battle gear. He looked with disdain upon the recruits who would, out of necessity, become his officers. His thin, black eyebrows crashed down on the bridge of his nose and the general's contempt hit his audience with such a force that many of them began to feel clammy sweat rising on their backs. Few could meet him eye to eye.

There were one hundred of Nanking's finest and best-educated youth in front of the general. The men were chosen to be officers because of their status and, most importantly, their ability to read and write. But status alone did not matter to General Kwan. Even the emperor's nephew could end up as a front-line infantry officer. As far as the general was concerned, a man's skill was the only thing that mattered. In a short time, each recruit would have to learn every aspect and position of the battlefield, starting from the basics up. Only their ability to master the different positions and skill levels would determine how high they rose in rank and position.

"Welcome to the Imperial Army!" General Kwan bellowed. "You are being trained to be my eyes, ears, and voice on the battlefield. I will depend upon you for victory."

Everyone roared approval, but General Kwan knew it was only the sound of naive bravado. He did not smile and his gaze turned even more fierce. The men quieted quickly.

"You have lived an easy life until now," he warned. "But I will force you to kill, to wear your enemy's blood upon you for days on end. You will be in an unimaginable hell. If you are strong of will and spirit, you *might* survive. If not, you will *die*!" The general paused. "It is that simple. Listen to your cadre, they will save your life."

The general's words called up Hunglu's feelings from the first attack upon his caravan so many years before, and the young man's first impression was that he should run. Perhaps better than any of the recruits around him, he could envision a hundred heads lying on the ground and nearly vomited at the thought. Yet, Hunglu allowed himself to quickly get caught up in the fervor of the group of young warriors-to-be. It was not long before he found himself cheering with the crowd.

Hunglu long idealized himself becoming as skilled a warrior as Cheng. The very thought fortified his resolve and summoned the hero within him to squelch his fears.

The recruits were broken up into squads of twenty each, with a seasoned captain supervising their training. The basic training began with strengthening exercises and beginning martial-arts techniques and stances. The men were forced to spend all instruction time in a horse-riding stance. There they remained for many painful hours, strengthening their legs and mental focus.

After the second day of training, Hunglu regretted having not regularly practiced his martial arts.

The next phase of basic training was learning how to fashion pikes—nine-foot poles with sharpened ends. Pikes were the basic weapon of front-line troops and were used to either stop cavalry or as a makeshift primitive spear. The front-line forces were really just a perimeter wall of defense, often referred to as the arrow catchers. They did not require much intelligence or training, but their role was vital on the battlefield. The officers of the front-line troops had to hold the line in order and maintain the courage of the other men under attack.

Spear training was the next level of skills the men needed to master. Spears could be up to eighteen-feet long, and the only difference between a spear and a pike was the cutting edge. The spear and the pole ax were used to cut and thrust with accuracy. There were six basic moves for the men to learn. The moves were then organized in various patterns to be practiced, mostly sparring with another recruit. Both ends of the spear were used as a weapon to strike, parry, and thrust. Spearmen were the main body of the forces and fought either mounted on horseback or on foot. Hunglu liked the spear very much. He quickly learned the weapon and already knew how *not* to attack a horseman from experience.

After spear training, the recruits were tested on their horse-riding skills to determine the best riders for cavalry training. Cavalry troops used the spear, cavalry sword, and the Kwando in battle, but most of the training was in the use of the horse as a battlefield weapon. Hunglu was not a good horseman, so he was quickly moved on to advanced infantry training.

Hunglu excelled in the tactics and use of the infantry's main weapon, the willow-leaf broadsword. The broadsword had a single-edged blade, twenty-eight to thirty-five inches in length. It was broader on the end than at the base, and had a curve that resembled the leaf of a willow tree. The strong sword was designed to be swung in wide circular patterns, hacking anything in its path. When sharp, the heavy steel sword effortlessly cut through bodies and armor. Even when dulled in battle, the sword became a deadly club. The massive weight of the sword gave it more power in the cut, and it was durable enough to survive years of impact. The broadsword also came in a long-handled version, where the sword was mounted on a three-foot handle. This weapon was versatile enough to fight hand-to-hand but was mostly designed to attack horses and their riders. Unlike the long and heavy Kwando, the long-handled broadsword was easily carried by slinging it over the back. Hunglu had to learn the basics of every weapon, including the Kwando.

The most powerful weapon, the bow and arrow, was reserved for the older warriors. Archers were selected from those who had archery experience, from seasoned warriors who had suffered limiting wounds, or from warriors who lacked physical endurance. A troop of archers could rain death down from the sky at over two hundred yards, decimating an advancing army. General Kwan recognized the power of archers on the battlefield. An archer could kill more men by luck than a skilled fighter employing great effort and tremendous risk.

The general intended to use archery to compensate for the Nanking-based army's lack of skill and experience.

One of General Kwan's innovations was to arm his cavalry with bows and swords rather than the traditional spears and Kwando. This innovation provided speed, mobility, and the ability to engage the enemy at a distance. The cavalry troops could charge in and rain arrows upon the front-line defenses before they could be engaged by the enemy archers themselves. Then they could withdraw and attack again from another direction, all this time providing cover for their advancing infantry troops. General Kwan wanted to break the enemy's defenses and morale with the least amount of risk to his men. But he also had some other innovations that, if successful, might end the war before it really began.

After four months of training, Hunglu had become skilled in warfare tactics, weapons, and battlefield philosophy. But the most important thing he learned was humility.

He was required to work as a team member and thus subjugate his will to his superiors for the success of the mission. He had been a man who walked with the most important members of the local government—men who had the emperor's ear. Now he was only a step higher than the quarry workers he had supervised. In construction he knew he had a future, ascending to higher positions; in his military training there were no such guarantees. Poor performance or insubordination meant commanding pikemen on the front line. Hunglu had no advantages available to him. He had to work, obey, and cooperate.

One day he was called out of formation by his captain. "The general wants you," was all he said.

Hunglu was instantly concerned.

After months of training to always expect the worst, and having watched the general in action, he was understandably nervous about this development. The general, in order to keep up his skills, routinely withdrew recruits to practice against. Hunglu had watched him beat five skilled recruits armed with broadswords in less than fifteen movements, using only a staff. The man who gave him the most trouble paid for it with a broken arm. Kwan was a demon incarnate.

With much trepidation Hunglu reported to the general's field tent. After three hours of waiting and worrying, he was given an audience.

"Hunglu, my officers have advised me that you excelled in your training," the general said with obvious approval. "This is good. You have earned the right to be one of my staff officers."

"Sir?"

The general leaned over his field desk, on which was a collection of hand-drawn rice-paper maps. "Your engineering skills and creativity are very much required by me. I have seen some of your bridges and the chapel at Shur's Grove. They are the products of a skilled intellect; therefore, I have decided to use your experience and your mind *here*, not on a battlefield."

"This army will traverse many obstacles and penetrate fortresses. We need a mind with an understanding of both military operations and structures to do this. I expect you to be able to use your existing knowledge of constructing buildings to aid us in destroying them more efficiently. Now report to Master Sun." The general waved a hand in the air, but did not turn to see Hunglu off.

Hunglu bowed to the general's back and did what he was told. He walked outside the tent and was met by a robust old man with a big grin.

"Ah, Hunglu, welcome to my service," Master Sun greeted him. "Come with me now."

Hunglu followed obediently. He was confused by this turn of events, yet deeply relieved that he would not be on the battlefield. But the sudden sense of relief shamed and embarrassed him; he had become friends with men who would lose their lives within minutes during an actual battle. His battlefield longevity as an infantry officer was also questionable. This reprieve from a near-certain death made him feel like a deserter. His mind rationalized that the decision was not his to make, that the general had intervened and orders were orders. Hunglu's heart, though, told him he was weak. He did not know how much danger he really was in.

MASTER SUN

Master Sun was an expert in fireworks, missiles, and explosives. Scars and pits in his body's flesh attested to the fact that this mastery was not easily won. But he was given the name Master Sun because he could light up the night with his flares and explosions for miles around. As they walked, Master Sun talked nonstop of what awaited Hunglu.

"We do not have much time," he said. "I must teach you all I know about explosives in just a few weeks."

"Why so quickly?"

"For your mission, of course," Master Sun answered.

"What mission?"

The old man grinned. "You will know that if you pass the training."

"What happens if I don't pass?" Hunglu asked cautiously.

"Then the birds will find pieces of you blown all through the trees." The old man laughed boldly. "You either succeed or you die, that's what war is about."

"Oh," Hunglu said.

It took two weeks for Hunglu to learn how to make bombs of various powers, how to mix powder, and how to time fuses. He learned about bomb placement and blast patterns. Each night he would return to his quarters with his clothes reeking of sulfur. His eyes burned and he ate his meals with blackened hands, yet the skills he was acquiring excited to him. Hunglu had always been fascinated by the New Year's fireworks in Nanking. The first time he saw them he was terrified at their noise and power. He had seen a stray rocket crash upon a roof and explode, destroying the upper floor of a building. Now he was learning how to precisely destroy whole buildings with the power of just that one rocket. He had spent a whole career learning how to keep buildings up, so it took very little time to learn how to break them down.

The trickiest part was timing the fuses for accurate, sequential blasts. To teach Hunglu the proper timing, Master Sun took him through many buildings in Nanking, placing fuses attached to small firecrackers in desirable locations. After few days of detailed study and practice, Hunglu was ready for field-testing. The old man and Hunglu traveled to a small abandoned temple. The walls, tinged with a thin layer of moss, were only twenty-feet high and the roof had sloughed off some its red tiles, but the pillars inside were still strong, the structure intact.

Master Sun directed Hunglu to look at the building and decide how to destroy it without anyone escaping. "You may observe the building for as long as you like. But you must finish the job quickly once you begin, and you must act without detection from any sentries," the old man said.

Hunglu did as he was told. He planned the operation for three hours in his mind. By then, it was growing dark, the sky fading behind charcoal-colored clouds. Hunglu sat from a position within the trees, staring and never removing his eyes from his objective. Finally he slipped into the shadows and moved stealthily toward the building.

Inside the temple halls, the air was sultry and reeked of decay. There was little light left coming through the shattered windows, but he did not need it; Hunglu knew this building as if he had built it himself and moved about it with ease. Rodents, snakes, and lizards were skittering and slithering around inside, roused by the moonlight. But Hunglu detected another presence and sensed that he was being watched. He knew that Master Sun might have entered the building to check his progress, but this presence felt much stronger than that of his teacher. He centered himself and refocused on his objective.

Hunglu had to place his explosives carefully. Even small variances in humidity levels from the time he placed the bombs until they actually exploded could affect the end result. The fuses were the most sensitive—any moisture at all would cause them to burn erratically. Hunglu had to remember the precise location for each of the twelve fist-sized bombs he set, for he could not go fumbling about trying to relocate them when fusing the whole building. Knowing where he was at all times was critical.

Hunglu emerged two hours later, the fuses lit and burning as he slinked away to a safe distance. He found Master Sun at the designated rendezvous point and neither said anything as they sat in anticipation.

The wait stretched out agonizingly for Hunglu. He second-guessed each of his bomb placements and the entire fuse layout. If he had made just one mistake, the whole effort might be lost. He was convinced that things had gone terribly wrong when the building suddenly erupted and fell into an inescapable pile of debris. Two weeks of playing with firecrackers and learning technical theory had not prepared him for the devastating force of high-powered explosives.

For a moment, Hunglu was blinded and deafened by the blast. His senses recoiled from overload and he felt a strange, yet somewhat familiar, sensation. It was as if he were about to be pulled into the sky by some incredible force. But most disconcerting was the fact that he thought that he heard someone call his name very clearly.

Then it was over, the light and the roar of the explosion. Hunglu's head was swimming, his eyes slowly adjusting to the night, his hearing dulled to the point where all sounds seemed as if they were coming through cotton wadding.

"You have passed your test!" Master Sun said proudly.

Hunglu could barely hear his master and pointed at his ears.

"Yes, I know! It will go away! There are still some things we must work on, but now we will eat and rest!" Master Sun grabbed Hunglu's black robe and pulled him into the brush.

Hunglu looked back. The crackling sound of the fire was beginning to filter through his ears and his vision was stabilizing. He wondered why the temple had been abandoned. Where were the men that once inhabited the walls he had just shattered? And what would they think if they one day returned and found their temple smashed, as if the thumb of some immortal master had simply pushed it into the ground. For a moment, Hunglu felt the senselessness of war. It was not natural. He was afraid to tell Master Sun for fear of what the old man might report to the general. Nor did Hunglu tell his master of the haunting voice he heard at the moment the building was destroyed. Instead, Hunglu pushed the regret from his mind and tried to revel in his achievement.

The farther into the woods they receded, the more the light and sound of the burning temple faded. Every few steps, Hunglu looked back. Finally all signs of great destruction disappeared, replaced by the ordinary sounds of the night and the glow of the moon. Hunglu again sensed that they were being watched by some entity, but his master did not seem to notice as he led the way through the thick trees. If Master Sun did not perceive another presence, neither would the pupil, Hunglu decided.

COMRADES

After two weeks of working nearly every hour of every day, words of praise from Master Sun were very welcome to Hunglu. He ate a big meal after his test and slept for half a day. They traveled back to the encampment at Nanking, and on the following day Hunglu was again in front of General Kwan and his senior staff.

"You have done well, and in a short time," the general said, now carefully appraising Hunglu. "Your talents have exceeded expectations."

Hunglu welcomed the general's approval and joy rose in his belly. He was careful, though, to appear serious and somber before this great man.

The general continued. "We have a most important mission for you. I want you to look at this map and listen to me closely . . ."

Hunglu plus four of Kwan's finest troops were to go into enemy-held territory and pinpoint the headquarters of the senior warlord for the rebel forces, a man named Lord Chu. In one month's time, Lord Chu was scheduled to attend a staff meeting with his generals and his southern ally, Lord Yang. Their objective was to convince one of the emperor's allies to defect. A senior allied general—Kwan did not know which—was to meet with the rebels, and it was Hunglu's mission to destroy the headquarters, Lord Chu, his generals, and the defector. Lord Chu's number-three general was willing to take control after the assassination. Then, left on his own, Lord Yang would either quickly cease conflict or be trapped between two strong armies. A great deal hinged on the success of Hunglu's team.

To ensure victory, General Kwan would lead his army south and east to attack the forces of Lord Yang. This assault would open a path to the southern borders and the sea. If Hunglu failed, the southern campaign would still landlock Lord Chu, cutting off his supplies and trade, but the imperial army would be at much greater risk. Lord Chu was likely to attack from the north and to the rear of the advancing imperial forces, eliminating a retreat and hammering them against the entrenched forces of Lord Yang. It was a very dangerous plan, but a good one. If successful, it would end the war before it really began. Hunglu felt the responsibility thrust upon him, yet his immediate concern was to figure out how he would get to the objective. And, he wondered, could five men possibly survive going into the heart of the enemy's territory? After the mission briefing, the general's staff introduced the other team members.

The leader of the group was Li, a Taoist from the Wu Tan mountains, who had been sent by his grandmaster to assist General Kwan in overthrowing the rebellion. He was a lean but strong man, about forty years in age and living the austere life of an ascetic monk. His sword was unusual—a thin two-handed, double-edged sword, which he wore slung over his back. He was a master of the internal Crane system of martial arts.

Li had much experience in leading these types of covert missions. On many occasions, monks from Wu Tan were requested to find and rescue hostages taken in an effort to acquire political favors. The monks' advanced martial training, mental focus, and total lack of regard for political allegiances made them excellent mercenaries. Li had tried for years to repress his warrior's heart and desire without success. Whenever a mission became available, his desires overrode his pacifist aspirations, forcing him to volunteer. His soul was that of a martial knight. Without hesitation, Li went wherever his services were requested.

Hou, their guide, was from the southeast territories where they were heading. Hou, like Lu, was a professional caravan guide, who at age thirty-four had already accumulated twenty-three years of professional guard experience. He escorted many caravans through this region and was very familiar with the areas they were traveling. He was an expert in his family's style of fighting, the Labyrinth. While proficient with all weapons, he preferred the simplicity of the willow-leaf broadsword. Conscripted to General Kwan's service because of his knowledge of the terrain and region, Hou was overjoyed to be of service, especially for this particular mission. Hou hated Lord Chu. On occasion, when the warlord's treasury was low, Chu attacked caravans for goods, sparing the guards if they remained quiet. For a small commission, nefarious escorts eventually started advising Chu which caravans were carrying the greatest valuables. Hou had escorted a caravan that was betrayed in this manner by a rival escort service. The caravan had been surrounded by an assault force of twenty of Lord Chu's cavalry, which was supported by ten archers. It would have been suicide to resist a professional military force of that strength, so Hou surrendered the caravan, along with his reputation. Now Hou wanted revenge for his loss of face. Guiding a team to kill Lord Chu would, in his mind, restore honor and fulfill his need for revenge.

Pi was an imperial guard from the forbidden city in Peking. He, as his father before him, was trained from childhood to serve and protect the emperor. At twenty-nine, he became a captain of the guard, chief instructor of martial arts, a master archer, and an expert at fortress defense and assault. His knowledge of booby traps was invaluable. Pi's loyalty to his emperor was religiously inspired: he believed in the divinity of his master and would do anything to protect the empire. Despite his intense beliefs, he was also a light-natured person who had a great sense of adventure. As skilled as Pi was, there was no opportunity within the forbidden city to practice his crafts. Essentially, his position was ceremonial, with no real opportunity to be an active martial knight. Pi was excited to be on the cusp of battle.

Yin was one of Kwan's lieutenant generals from the northern provinces. He was tall and muscular, with an intimidating presence and attitude. Trained by his father, he was a practitioner of the long-fist fighting style and a master of the double-edged sword. At thirty, he was Kwan's youngest general.

Yin had trained and fought under General Kwan for eight years, and was furious that Kwan had appointed a monk to lead a combat expedition deep into enemy territory. Yin hated the mission, but his obedience to his commander was a matter of honor, and he suppressed his objections. It was obvious, though, that he looked at his teammates with contempt, especially Hunglu, the most inexperienced of them all.

But once Hunglu met his team members, he felt more confident. The group of four men was equivalent to a force of forty. Now all they had to worry about was moving explosives one hundred miles in two weeks without being detected by enemy troops.

There was little time to prepare, and the next day the five warriors carefully packed as many explosives as they could, loaded the

67

ordinance on horses, and were off. They had to move quickly, but also avoid detection or any engagement with enemy forces.

Li was a very quiet leader, speaking only when necessary. It was clear that he was keenly observant. Though Yin did not cause any direct problems, it soon became obvious to all through his actions that he hated being there. Hunglu was concerned that perhaps Yin would try to assume command from Li and a duel would ensue. Li showed no recognition that a problem even existed, he just politely instructed them what to do and everyone did it. Yin, in spite of his resistance, could not help but voluntarily comply.

On the third day of the expedition, the small demolition force had crossed the border between their own defenses and Lord Chu's territory. That evening they set up camp in the midst of a dense forest and sat quietly around a small, smokeless fire. The spring air was still cold and damp. Hunglu felt his body fill with tremors and hoped it would not lead to sickness.

Li addressed the group after they had eaten. "It is absolutely essential that we move undetected through the areas ahead," he said. "Hou, you and Hunglu pick the safest, quickest, most undetectable course of travel . . ."

Hunglu had assumed he would be involved with deciding the safest path for the volatile explosives, but Li's next words shocked him.

"Hunglu, use your flying spirit to find us the safest routes to travel. You will describe them to Hou, and he will guide us to those trails. Only your spirit can tell us where the enemy lies." Li spoke in a matter-of-fact tone and the others seemed to accept his declaration without question.

But Hunglu didn't understand. "I . . . I can't do that. That's an impossible thing to ask of me!" he stuttered.

All eyes were suddenly upon Hunglu.

It was Yin who spoke: "The boy will get us all killed." His voice was gruff and contemptuous.

"No," Li said. "He has the skill. He simply lacks technique, which I will teach him."

"He has no confidence," Yin countered. "He will get nervous and fail. Look at him." Yin pointed to Hunglu, shaking beneath a rough, wool blanket.

"He will gain confidence with practice," Li said.

"I've never done anything like this before!" Hunglu protested. Already he felt the tension of this new responsibility adding pressure to his overburdened mind. This hadn't been part of the assignment.

"Hunglu may doubt himself as a man," Li began, "and he may doubt his abilities to accomplish what is asked of him. And it is true that I, too, doubt his ability as an inexperienced man, *but* I do not doubt his spirit's ability to *make* him succeed, in spite of doubts and fears. You see, Yin, he will succeed because it is his destiny. The immortals have already decided this."

Hunglu admitted to the others that he could only remember a few times in his life when he consciously chose to travel to a particular place, and even then he had achieved only mixed results. He certainly did not want the lives of four comrades and an invading army depending upon his dreams.

Yin was incredulous. With a horrid expression, he made it clear he wasn't going to easily put his life into the hands of an inexperienced soldier using foolish mysticism. Now he resented even more that General Kwan had appointed this scrawny monk command over him.

"This is beyond belief!" Yin scoffed, further shaking Hunglu's confidence. "I will have no part of this nonsense!"

Li spoke calmly to Yin. "I understand your concerns, and you don't have to be a part of this nonsense, as you call it. You are free to go back if you do not wish to follow commands. But you must choose, Yin. If you stay you must never doubt this man or his abilities, and if you go you must leave now."

Hou sat expressionless, unwilling or unable to say anything. Pi, on the other hand, was excited; he had seen oracles predict many events that came to pass.

All the men knew that Li was not offering Yin much of a choice. If Yin left, General Kwan would have his head upon a pole. But if he stayed his head would probably end up on Lord Chu's pole instead. At least with the latter he had the opportunity of taking a few of the enemy with him and would die with honor. The wild card was that Yin could choose to defect to the enemy. It was a heavy wager Li was making, and the other men knew it: Li was relying entirely on Yin's sense of duty.

A silent battle ensued, lasting nearly an hour, during which none of the men spoke and Li and Yin gazed at each other over the fire.

Each was looking into the other's eyes in search of weakness and a lack of resolve.

"I will stay and honor my position," Yin finally said.

Li leaned forward. "Very good, Yin. It is unlikely we would have succeeded without you." Then he made Hunglu leave the fire for a moment so he could speak to the other men. When Hunglu returned, Li guided him into the woods.

FLYING SPIRIT

Away from the light of the fire, Hunglu could only see the silhouette of Li at his side. The chill was intense, and the moon was hooked into the black night like a shard of ice. They walked for a long time and were far from the fire before Li began to talk.

"Hunglu, I will teach you the seeing techniques that you will need to know, but, above all, do not be afraid of failing. If you fear failure you will create it for yourself," Li cautioned. "You will most likely make mistakes, and some of them will be dangerous, but that is nothing to fear. If you make a mistake, we have the resources and skills to survive and still succeed in our mission."

Hunglu was comforted by Li's confidence in the success of the mission.

"Now sit over here and rest against the tree," Li directed, then waited a moment before continuing. "Until this moment, you have used your abilities without focus and have gotten mixed results. This has not helped your confidence in those abilities. Now we will train you to wield your mind like a sword—with accuracy and precision. Start to concentrate on your breathing, and with each breath relax your body so that you become as soft as cotton."

Li let Hunglu relax for a few minutes before going on.

"Hunglu, I want you to create a sacred space in your mind, a peaceful place, a place that you may have visited in real life. Tell me when you see this place around you."

"I see it," Hunglu said, visualizing a hilltop within his mind. The hilltop overlooked a valley, but he had never been there before. There were posts and stones planted in the ground. The configuration of the area was odd, but the peacefulness and familiarity of the setting soothed him. He suddenly realized that he was no longer cold.

"Good," Li continued, "now imagine a bag of salt in your hand. Draw a large circle of salt upon the ground of that place, surrounding your body."

In Hunglu's mind he made the circle around him, surprised that there was truly a bag of salt in his hand to begin with.

Li's voice became more quiet. "Now sit in the circle and concentrate on breathing. Be the person in the circle, *be* in that place. Look out in the distance of that place and feel your breath in that body, forgetting you are here . . ."

Hunglu felt his body on the hill becoming more and more real, until it was the only body he had ever had.

". . .Feel your soul within you, within your heart. Feel it becoming a sun, a brilliant sun within you. . ."

Hunglu heard Li's voice in the center of his head, and there was a gentle heat rising inside his chest. The heat slowly became a force of energy radiating outward.

". . .Let your body become the sun. . ."

Hunglu felt his body becoming a ball of energy as he slowly rose up from the ground.

". . .Hou, Pi, and Yin have hidden three objects in the forest. Find them and describe them to me . . ."

Hunglu's spirit eyes searched the dark forest as he flew above the treetops. It was not long before he sensed a square gold object shining out from under some pine needles. Concentrating on this spot, he saw a belt buckle. It looked like Hou's. Hunglu described it to Li and where it was located.

The next thing Hunglu was drawn to was a tree limb. He didn't know why he was attracted to it, so he floated around the limb for a long time. Finally, he discovered that there was a coin nestled in the crook of a branch. Hunglu knew that coin belonged to Pi because he could see the imperial seal.

Excited, Hunglu turned his attentions to finding what Yin had left. He saw Yin walking out of the forest alone. Hunglu was drawn to a group of wild flowers, particularly a yellow one, but he could not find anything that Yin left, no matter how hard he looked. He told this to Li.

". . .Good, Hunglu . . . now come back to your circle. Move back into your body . . . feel your living body breathing. Feel yourself firmly on the ground."

Hunglu felt himself again resting upon the tree and opened his eyes. "That was so real," he said. "It was like I was there! But I'm sorry I couldn't find what Yin left."

"That's fine, you did very well." Li suspected trickery on Yin's part. "Let's go and find out how well you really did."

As they walked back to the camp Li told Hunglu more about viewing things from a distance. He stressed that the meditation technique was just a training tool; Hunglu could quickly learn to view while walking or doing any daily activity. Then he warned Hunglu, "The one thing you must never do, is assume you know what you are looking at."

"What do you mean?" asked Hunglu.

"If you see tree bark, do not assume it is attached to a tree. It may be the siding of a house, a pile of logs, a constructed box, or even scaffolding for a building. If you see the bark *and* the tree, only then is it a tree."

Hunglu wondered why the team was not being led by Li's vision and asked as much.

"You have the ability to fly with your spirit, I can only see with mine," Li explained.

Hunglu shook his head. "I don't understand."

"Imagine that we are both trying to see a far off mountain. I can see the mountain as if it is a painting, but you have the ability to fly and follow a path to the mountain. For this mission, it is very important that we see an accurate path. It is a minor difference in ability, but a major difference as far as *this* mission is concerned. We cannot afford to miss a single sentry," Li said solemnly. "And with you guiding us, I can focus objectively upon the mission rather than being tainted by my emotions to support my visions."

Hunglu did not know what to say and remained silent. Tainted by emotions supporting the visions? What did Li mean? Hunglu was excited about his newfound gift, but Li spoke of emotions as if they were something beyond his control. Hunglu looked at Li as they walked back to the camp, but the thin monk said nothing. The air was still and Hunglu suddenly felt the vastness of the woods around him. It was a lonely place, even with companions. A sudden sense of profound isolation absorbed him. He looked up through the gaps between the trees. All signs of the moon were gone and what lay beyond were cold, distant stars, each separated from the others by vast distances.

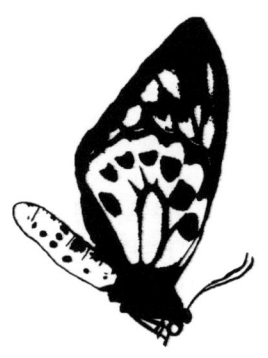

THE PLAN

Hunglu and Li met the others back at the camp. The three men were sitting around the dying fire, quietly murmuring to each other. Li and Hunglu were almost upon them before the other men even knew, and for a moment Hunglu wondered if they were still traveling in spirit form.

Pi and Hou were very impressed at the accuracy Hunglu demonstrated with his descriptions. But then Hunglu admitted to Yin that he could not find what the warrior left.

"I saw you in the forest," Hunglu said. "And I saw a yellow flower, but could not find anything you hid for me."

Yin turned red with embarrassment and amazement. "I peed on that flower," Yin said, beginning to laugh. "I left you pee to find, Hunglu!"

The others all laughed and Yin slapped Hunglu on the back, nearly bringing the young man to his knees.

"Hunglu, if you can find my pee in the forest, then I can follow your visions," Yin said.

With their tensions waning, the men in the demolition party rested for the serious journey ahead.

Hunglu's visions proved flawless in finding the best routes to the site. He even found water and rations for the small force along the way. This further impressed Yin, who was growing fonder of Hunglu with each passing day. Sometimes the two would walk ahead or behind the others, talking for hours. Yin wanted to know how to access his own powers of vision. Hunglu explained it as best he could, and sometimes Yin would make comical attempts, his face turning red and eyes bulging as he tried to push his spirit from his body by brute force.

The small imperial force arrived outside the defensive perimeter of Lord Chu's headquarters ten days later. After finding a suitable campsite, they set to work on their objectives.

Hunglu sized up the main structure while Yin and Pi assessed the defenses. The team came together with a plan. The main headquarters could be destroyed by setting multiple charges outside the walls and inserting a single large interior bomb on a roof beam. The exterior ordinance would destabilize the base of the walls, leaving the internal bomb and gravity to do the rest. If the plan was correct, the building would drop into rubble. Backing up the primary plan, it was decided that incendiary bombs would be used to set the rubble on fire, preventing any rescue attempts and finishing off the survivors. Hunglu reasoned that only someone protected by the immortals would be able to survive.

It was Pi's task to develop an entry plan, while Yin developed a method of escape. When they were all in agreement, the men chose to place the charges the next day, then on the day of attack they would set the fuses and finish the job. Heavily camouflaged in mud and leaves, they went to sleep, dreaming of the dangerous job ahead.

During the night Hunglu had a disturbing vision of another temple built into a mountain. It had only a single front wall—the rest was built into the mountain, making it inaccessible. In the dream, he did not see anyone enter or leave the temple, but Hunglu sensed that the second temple was where the actual meeting would take place. He woke with a shock and told the other members of the team.

"Our spies must have been wrong!" Yin whispered fiercely after hearing the news.

"Or, perhaps *their* spies heard of the plot," Pi suggested.
Li was pensive.

Hou had confirmed the existence of the temple; it was another day's journey away. "What should we do?" he asked.

"General Kwan has ordered us to destroy the headquarters," Yin said with resolve.

"Yes," Li agreed, "we must do that. But our mission also requires that we destroy Lord Chu. We will see what we can do . . . come with me, Hunglu."

The men started to rise.

"Wait here," Li commanded, shooting the men a stern look that none of them had seen before.

When Li and Hunglu were a good distance from camp, Li stopped beside a tree, put a hand on Hunglu's shoulder, and looked him straight in the eyes.

"Are you *sure* of your vision, Hunglu?" Li asked carefully.

Not since Yin, on the third night of the expedition, had anyone questioned his visions, and now Li himself was questioning him. Hunglu was about to question himself when he heard himself reply with total conviction: "Yes, I am certain."

Tension eased from Li's face.

"We will try finding out what's going on."

"How?" Hunglu asked.

"We will go into meditation together, and I'll follow you to the temple. Adding my perceptions with yours, we will confirm the truth." Li sat down and assumed a meditative posture. "Let your spirit meet me at the top of this tree."

Hunglu sat at the base of the tree and went into his meditation process, floating upward out of his body. At the top of the tree he saw a luminescent being that resembled Li, but it looked less human, less human even than himself.

"Go to the temple," Li said.

Hunglu heard the words inside him, almost as if they were his own thoughts. Li reached out and held him, but not with a hand; Hunglu felt Li's guidance as intention and *will*. It was a strange sensation, like a mixture of Hunglu's mind and Li's working together, making Hunglu feel stronger than ever before.

They were at the temple very quickly, and it was immediately clear to Li that this was a very different situation.

"What room did you see them in?" Li asked, trying to get more details.

"I didn't *see* them."

That wasn't the answer Li wanted. "Then we must go forward in time," he said. "Think about the day when Lord Chu will be here, and hold on to me with your thoughts."

Hunglu focused on two days into the future. He heard horses in the distance, a gentle sound at first, then growing in power to a thundering roar. Li and Hunglu looked over to the west and saw Lord Chu and the generals approaching. They galloped to the temple gate, dismounted, and entered the side of the mountain.

"Hold them in your mind and follow where they go," Li instructed.

Hunglu passed through the thick walls of the temple and found himself and Li in the main room of the temple. They heard small bits of talk: the number-three general had been killed for treason. Troops were being aligned along the emperor's borders. Victory would be swift, Chu and his comrades believed.

"Hunglu, memorize the room and examined it for an attack," Li commanded.

When Hunglu examined the structures and went inside the walls, he discovered an air-vent system over the temple room. The main airshaft went up through the mountain and into a clearing. Then, being careful to take Li with him, Hunglu flew over the mountain to find a route to the airshaft opening.

Li requested a survey of the defenses in and around the mountain. This took better than two hours. It seemed that at almost every turn there was some obstacle with which to contend. Lord Chu, was not a stupid man, and there were very few weaknesses in the mountain stronghold. Li and Hunglu double-checked all their observations. Satisfied that they had all the information they could gather, the two astral spies returned to their bodies under the tree.

"We will have to adjust our plans," Li decided.

It took them a few minutes to reorient themselves. Once they were fully back into their bodies, they quietly walked through the woods to rejoin the group.

Yin, Hou, and Pi had busied themselves with preparing the bombs. They did this at a great distance from each other, hunched over their work like mothers protecting infants. Should there be an accident, the others would at least be out of harm's way. Li called them back to the main encampment.

"We will have to divide the group and make two coordinated attacks," Li said. "Yin and I will destroy the headquarters, as per the original plan. Hunglu will place the charges, at which point we will infiltrate and hold our positions until the general's staff meeting. Yin and I will then set the fuses and follow Yin's escape plan. This is the place where we will most likely have to battle our way out." Li drew a crude map of the temple's interior and pointed toward a point near the main entrance.

Yin nodded in approval at the monk's plan.

"Hunglu, after you set the charges, you and Pi will go to the temple and infiltrate through the air vents. When Lord Chu enters and begins his meeting you will use your explosives and kill them. Your only escape is back through the shaft. From there you will be on your own."

"Hou will take the horses and supplies and wait at the safe meeting place by the stream located between the two attack sites. It is far and you will have to hurry."

Li finished his directions by allowing each team only two days to reach the meeting place. Otherwise, they would be assumed dead.

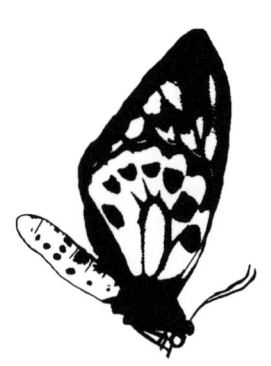

THE ATTACK

The operation began in the middle of the night. Most high-level headquarters had the luxury of an internal sewage system so the officials would not have to inconvenience themselves in bad weather. A drainage ditch would run under the complex from the main headquarters. Pi knew that the drainage ditch would have an unguarded fence at the end and that there would be at least one open area close to a sentry station. Pi also knew from experience that, because of the smell and improbability of infiltration, most sentries ignored the ditch.

Yin, Pi, Li, and Hunglu crawled quietly through the sewage ditch. They had stuffed pieces of rags scented with rose water up their nose. The ground beneath their feet was slick, and there was no way to convince themselves that they were traipsing through a less-noxious substance. Of more concern, though, was keeping the explosives from coming in contact with any moisture. It took the demolition party an hour to reach the center of the compound. At the end of their journey, they slipped into the small opening between building's foundation and the first floor. From here on out, they would be watching for snakes in addition to the other dangers that lurked above.

Positioning the explosives was tricky. Hunglu and Pi crawled very quietly under the floorboards of the headquarters, setting charges and laying fuse lines around the perimeter of the building. Yin climbed out of the latrine and into the building. Hunglu had instructed him to set two charges on the main roof beam. These charges could not be set off with fuses. Directly beneath the beam, Hunglu loosened some floorboards and rigged a special explosive that would launch upward like a flaming rocket. The white-hot magnesium would set off the beam charges, collapsing the flaming roof down upon the enemy. It took until dawn to complete the setup.

Pi and Hunglu barely got away from the compound before sunrise. Yin and Li sat quietly in the latrine for the next day and a half, waiting until they could light the fuses. Hunglu wondered what interesting things they were thinking, especially Yin, who had urinated on a flower in the not-so-distant past. Now Yin would know how it felt.

Pi and Hunglu traveled toward the meeting place with Hou for a half-day, then the rest of the way to the temple by themselves. They were able to find the access to the airshaft and slip into it with hours to spare.

The plan was simple. A table for the meeting had been set up about twenty feet from the altar. The airshaft ended at an opening in the fifteen-foot-high ceiling and was centered between the altar and the table. It was from there that the first bomb would drop.

Hunglu had made a special explosive with steel balls in it to kill the people at the meeting. The fuse was set so that the bomb would explode just as it hit the floor, and the blast was designed to go up to chest level. The front wall would direct more blast back to the targets, but the stone structure of the temple would remain undamaged. Hunglu planned for himself and Pi to be positioned in perpendicular sub-shafts when the bomb was dropped. This was the only way they could be protected from the fiery air blasting upward.

Rigging the headquarters had taken almost all of the explosive powder and there was only enough left for two small bombs. Hunglu had one bomb with him and a second bomb outside the building, should they need it for their escape. They could not bring the second bomb into the shaft because the blast from the first might set off the second, creating too much heat for Pi and Hunglu to survive. They only had one opportunity, so Hunglu triple-checked everything and rehearsed exactly how he would do it. He would light the fuse, drop the bomb, watch it until it exploded, and move his head back into the side shaft as soon as he saw a flash. Until Lord Chu arrived, Hunglu compulsively reviewed the steps he had laid out for himself, programming his body to act precisely. There was only one chance.

Hunglu and Pi knew that Lord Chu was in the building long before he entered the chamber. They heard a great deal of excited chatter echoing in the shafts from various rooms. Finally, their quarry burst into the room.

Lord Chu was an angry man it seemed. He paced about the room like a nervous animal and yelled about a number of things that were not to his liking. Hunglu could not see the lord's face, but the red garbs he wore flowed behind him like flames. As Hunglu checked the bomb one last time, he wondered why a man like Lord Chu, who appeared so unhappy with his current state, would desire more power. In the corner of his eye, he saw Pi signal across the gap between the airshafts. Pi held up one finger and winked. Hunglu nodded back.

To eliminate any obstructions between the bomb and the primary targets, Hunglu and Pi waited until all the guards left. Then Hunglu struck a powder-covered stick and ignited an oil cord. Using the cord like a candle, he lit the fuse, looked at Pi, and dropped the bomb.

To Hunglu the bomb appeared to fall in slow motion. He watched it descend and hit the floor. And then, to his horror, he saw the fuse pop out on impact.

No explosion.

"What's that?" Lord Chu suddenly called out. "Guards!"

Hunglu did not think. He focused on the bomb and dropped the fifteen feet to the granite floor as guards rushed into the room. In an instant, he stuck the flaming oil cord into the fuse hole and tossed the bomb into the air, covering his ears and head.

Pi saw Hunglu jump and looked down to see his comrade shuffling with bomb parts. A moment later, Pi's vision was obscured by a blinding flash of light. He barely pulled his head back before the super-heated air rushed past his face, singeing his short beard.

As Hunglu had planned, the blast went over his head. However, he had not planned that the heat would pull all the air out of his lungs, burn the clothes off his back, and grind him flat into the floor like a giant stepping on his back. Hunglu was crushed into unconsciousness.

Ringing becomes a roar. He is being hurled through the walls. . . the men in the room die . . . their souls are ripped from their bodies . . . their bodies disintegrate . . . their surprise. . .their horror. . .his horror. . .

One guard running into the room did not take a fatal blast; instead he died slowly from his wounds, in burning agony.

Hunglu was looking at a room full of spirits no different than he. They started to become dull in appearance as the shock and reality of their death set in. He saw one of the spirits start to turn inward upon itself, becoming encased in darkness, like in a small box. Another stumbled around cursing, grabbing at body parts, and finally ran out of the room. The others stood still, as if afraid to move. They could only look around at the walls covered with splashes of blood and flecks of human skin and bone. There was the sickening smell of burning hair filling the air.

It was not long before bright people, like lights, came down for each one of the dead and guided them away from the room. Hunglu watched for a long time until he was inextricably drawn to his own bright light coming from the wall. He walked to meet it and suddenly found himself in a garden with his father and mother.

"Father, what are you doing here?"

Hungling came over and embraced his son. "I died this past spring, Hunglu."

Hunglu noticed that his mother and father both appeared much younger than when he had known them as a child. His grandparents were there, too. They also appeared younger.

"Hunglu, you can't stay here, you will have to leave. But we will meet and journey together again," his mother told him. "You are here for another reason. You are to meet someone very important. Listen to what he has to tell you, my son."

"I want to stay with you," Hunglu said.

Hunglu felt someone touch his shoulder, he turned and saw a very bright being greeting him.

"Hello, Flying Spirit, I will be your teacher for the years to come, but you have not yet fulfilled your purpose in life. Be strong, you will not die today."

Hunglu did not know that resisting life would be harder than resisting death. He wanted to stay, but he felt his spirit being forced gently and firmly back into the blackness, the pain.

Hunglu gasped, feeling the incredible agony of his burned skin and crushed back.

"You succeeded, Hunglu. You are a hero," Pi whispered. He wanted Hunglu to know this before he died.

Hunglu coughed a ragged, unintelligible response. Pi did not know how to handle his friend. The entire backside of Hunglu had been damaged beyond any degree Pi had ever seen and enormous blisters were growing as he watched. Even what was left of Hunglu's black hair appeared melted to his scalp.

More guards were rushing down the hallways as Hunglu again lapsed into unconsciousness. Pi quickly pulled out a ceremonial dagger and put it to Hunglu's throat. It would be a far more honorable death than being left to the enemy, an enemy that would feed the last scraps of life in Hunglu to their dogs. He was ready to sink the knife into the crevasse just beneath Hunglu's jaw line when Hunglu struggled. Pi held him tighter, but Hunglu's protests grew more agitated. Pi did not know where his wounded friend's strength was coming from and suspected that it was divinely inspired.

He hoped that the Buddhists, being consistent in their temple designs, would have an emergency exit by the altar. Though not in the original escape plan, Pi found the panel to the left of the altar and stuffed Hunglu and himself through the doorway, getting it closed just before the guards entered the room. If luck was with them, no one would know about the door. Pi drew his sword and silently waited, listening to the mass confusion.

"Close the temple! Find who did this!" cried out a voice.

The guards left the room in search of the killers. Pi dragged Hunglu down the secret hallway and up a hundred steps to an exit on top of the mountain. Pi, who was scorched and exhausted himself, retched at the smell of Hunglu's still-smoldering flesh. He realized that Hunglu would not live, but Pi was determined to do everything possible to help him.

Miles away, Chu's headquarter's building exploded into rubble. The firebombs followed on time, setting it ablaze. The force of the explosion and flames was so great that all the soldiers outside were shocked into immobility. Li and Yin were able to walk right out of the compound during the confusion, as if they belonged there. Everyone else was running in all directions.

Many of the superstitious troops assumed that demons had destroyed the headquarters and began deserting their posts *en masse.*

As they walked away from the compound, Yin was amazed at how well the plan had worked. General Kwan was brilliant, he thought. Yin did not yet know about Hunglu's wounds.

Li, on the other hand, had a feeling that Hunglu was in danger. Since the beginning, Li had had reservations about sending inexperienced soldiers on such an important mission. His intuition had led him to believe the team would be successful, but there had also been a gray uneasiness that haunted him. Now his intuition was speaking clearly. Although his eyes were looking straight ahead, Li's mind could see Pi frantically hauling Hunglu's limp body up the dark and dank stairway. He could see the oozing wounds and knew how little time stood between Hunglu and death.

"We have to go to Hunglu," Li said.

The men stole two horses still tied to posts outside the compound and rode off.

ESCAPE

It had taken Pi half a day to carry Hunglu down the mountain. He had to be alert to patrols that were combing the mountainside, limiting the speed at which he could travel. Hunglu drifted in and out of delirium, and several times he nearly gave away their position with rants about a water well and death and lights.

Pi again heard horses approaching and hid, covering Hunglu's mouth with his hand. Pi could feel a warm dewy wetness soaking through his shirt as Hunglu was pressed against him. He hoped that Hunglu would not wake up and begin shrieking.

Li had been like a man possessed, focused only on finding Hunglu and Pi. He and Yin had ridden hard for hours and now his senses were drawn to a set of bushes.

Peering out from the brush, Pi yelled, "Li! Over here!"

Yin located the voice and pointed Pi and Hunglu out to Li who already had them in his sight. They rode quickly to the bushes and dismounted.

Li saw the burns on Pi's face first, then he saw the damage to Hunglu. He set to work, quickly removing Hunglu's dead skin and gave orders to Pi and Yin to gather medicinal herbs and leaves. The men went off quickly to accomplish their assigned tasks. Pi gathered the nearby leaves while Yin mounted his horse and rode up the mountain to where the herbs Li desired could be found. For the first time, Yin forgot he was at war, an error that led him into an enemy patrol.

"Stop! Stop!" an officer with a Kwando commanded.

There were only five soldiers, four of them with swords. Yin could simply ride off, but then they would alert the rest of the troops. No, he would have to kill them.

"I surrender!" Yin shouted, then dismounted.

All the men in the patrol had drawn their swords and surrounded him.

"Lay down your weapon!" the officer commanded.

Yin made every effort to appear as if he would comply legitimately, and no one saw what came next. He withdrew his sword and took the head of the nearest soldier to the rear—there wasn't even time for the victim to gasp in surprise. With the same stroke Yin pivoted his body, cutting the sword arm off the second rear swordsman. A back flick of his wrist cut the man's throat. Then he took two steps forward and his thrust entered the next swordsman's heart. At the same time the last swordsman swung his broadsword in an attempt to split Yin's head. Yin quickly stepped inside the blow, undercut the man's wrist, and smashed the spiked pummel of his sword into the man's skull. Now he squared himself before the officer, who had not moved.

"I am Chu Wushan," the large man said coldly. "I will now avenge my father's death!"

Chu's son, how noble, Yin thought. "I am General Yin of the Imperial Army of Nanking! You need not die for your father's honor."

"So the devil dog Kwan is behind all this," Chu spat. "I shall send him your head!"

Chu moved fast, thrusting his blade and then slashing upward and over with the blade and pole point.

Yin stayed out of range of the long weapon. It was clear that Chu had mastered this weapon, but, fortunately, Yin had spent many hours fighting with the Grandmaster Kwan himself. He evaded Chu's attacks with footwork, knowing the only defense against the Kwando was to not be there when it struck.

His strategy was to out maneuver Chu into overextending himself, thus creating an opening for a counterattack. Yin backed himself up a small hill to get Chu off balance. As Chu furiously advanced up hill, Yin quickly moved down and faked a thrust, causing Chu to swing awkwardly. This action succeeded in making Chu lose his balance. Yin stepped quickly into Chu's center and wheeled his sword over his right shoulder, slashing down upon Chu's neck, severing his arteries and windpipe.

Dying now, Chu slashed upward with the point end of the Kwando, breaking one of Yin's left ribs. Chu then followed with a crossing strike toward Yin's head. It was the last move Chu made.

Yin checked the sweeping blow with his sword and kicked Chu's knee, buckling his leg. Chu crumpled forward upon Yin's legs, pinning him to the ground. Freeing his sword as he fell, Yin executed a slide cut across Chu's neck. There was a gush of blood, a final gasp of the enemy, and the fight was over.

Yin painfully untangled himself from Chu's body, feeling the penalty for his overconfidence and underestimation of Chu. But now he had to put his pain and anger aside to find the herbs that would save Hunglu's life. He took a piece of white-willow bark from his pouch and chewed it to help with the pain. An hour later, Yin had collected and delivered the herbs to Li.

"What happened?" Pi asked, while Li worked on Hunglu.

"I foolishly forgot where I was," Yin growled and showed Pi the massive bruise on his side.

"Come here and let me fix that," Pi said. He tore some strips of fabric from Yin's shirt and tied them around his ribcage, splinting the broken section as much as possible.

As Pi worked on him, Yin sat back and looked at Hunglu's near-dead body. Yin had seen many battles and dying men. He knew that Li would pull Hunglu out of this crisis, but more importantly he knew Hunglu had the spirit to pull himself from death's claws. Then Yin looked away: these men with whom he fought had taught him a new level of camaraderie and given him a vision of an era of magical warfare that could change the world forever. Yin would return to General Kwan as a reinvented soldier, and perhaps, Yin thought, that was what Kwan might have had on his mind all along.

Li prepared a poultice and placed it on Hunglu's back to prevent infection and stimulate healing. Hunglu's bandages were constructed from gingko leaves, but despite his best efforts, Li knew it was essential to get Hunglu to a monastery for medical treatment. Only Hou would know where the nearest one could be found and the men quickly packaged Hunglu for travel to the rendezvous point.

Hou guided the soldiers to the Gateway to Heaven Monastery, a three-day journey to the north. None of them talked much as they followed trails by night to avoid detection. Sometimes they listened as Hunglu, slung over a horse, prattled on about water wells and death and his mother and father. The men were unable to discern any meaning from what they heard.

Every day, the group found a small cave or dense brush in which to hide. Li removed Hunglu's dead skin and reapplied fresh poultices and gingko bandages. During this time, Hunglu would nearly surface from his dreams and whimper sadly. He did not scream, and for that, Li was thankful. He knew that if Hunglu were to become fully conscious, he would feel the brunt of the pain with such force that he might never stop screaming. If that happened, Li knew that Hunglu would beg to be put out of his misery. Li also knew that they might have to obey such a wish and commend Hunglu to the immortals. As it was, Hunglu did not wake up. He grew more quiet with every passing hour. Near the end of the journey, he went silent, and the men tramped on in the night, the soft clopping of the horses filling the emptiness. Each was afraid to check on their companion for fear of discovering that he was dead.

The Grandmaster of the temple was not surprised to see soldiers arrive at the front gates. He provided them with food, lodging, and took over the care of Hunglu. The temple physician continued to give Hunglu a regiment of herbs, but warned Li, Yin, Pi, and Hou not to expect Hunglu to live much longer. All of the men were hidden within the temple so that renegade enemy forces looking for revenge would not be able to find the small demolition team. The five men were so well concealed that many of the monks in the compound did not even know of their existence.

A week after they arrived, the four warriors had recovered their strength enough to continue. Li decided that they needed to finish their mission. They left Hunglu at the monastery early one morning and headed south to join General Kwan's army.

Hunglu didn't regain consciousness until days after they departed. The physician brought Hunglu a gift Yin left: it was a gold medallion that was given to Yin by General Kwan. The physician explained that were it not for the talents and courage of Hunglu, the demolition team would never have achieved its objectives, and perhaps the empire would have fallen. Each time he looked at the medal, Hunglu lamented the fact that he was never able to tell his friends goodbye. In the end, he simply wrapped it in rice paper and put it away from his sight.

His healing took a long time, and after weeks in bed Hunglu had become frail, unable to even walk across the room without help from the physician. The physician often said prayers as he helped Hunglu to convalesce. At first, Hunglu didn't pay much attention, but slowly the prayers became an integral part of his routine, and he found himself repeating the words by rote memory. Certain prayers seemed to have more power than the others, and Hunglu began to recite them even when the doctor was not around. In moments of great pain, he whispered the words over and over, focusing on their cadence. In this way he was able to soothe himself. Other times he could hear the sound of prayer drifting from the temple, and Hunglu, alone, would chant the words with the monks. He hoped that somewhere, Li, Pi, Hou, and Yin could hear him.

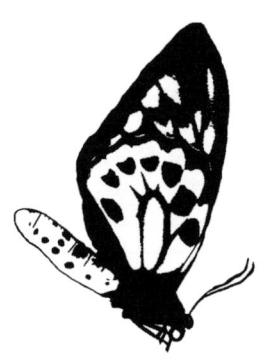

THE SWORD OF THE MIND

The sunset was beautiful on the west side of the mountain. The sinking sun cast off layers of orange and red, like sheets of silk. Hunglu rooted himself to the ground and faced his back to the rising night sky. Feeling his feet equally weighted, he allowed all the muscles in his legs and buttocks to relax. He then practiced breathing as before.

The colors in the sky intensified as he became more and more serene in his stance. He felt as if he had no body. Slowly, the colors of the sunset permeated his soul. It was a profound feeling. The various hues of red and orange brought vitality into him, a vitality that was lacking after all his mental reviews. Here again the Grandmaster was correct: if one spent too much time focusing on the past, it took the Chi away from the body.

Hunglu continued to recharge.

The parrot left the pouch, climbed up Hunglu's shirt, and stood on his shoulder. There, it began to watch the sunset too, calling out, *Braaahahahah.... heeeehaaahaha...oooohahooho*!

Startled from his meditation, Hunglu could not help laughing at the bird's absurd noises. If a bird has to learn only one thing from man, he thought, then it should learn laughter.

Hunglu and the parrot walked home in the fading light, Hunglu gathering fresh pine nuts and berries for the parrot's evening meal. The bird was very interested in these foraging activities and flew to the ground where it did a lot of squawking, moving, chewing, and just playing. Whenever its master walked away, the bird would stop and fix its eye upon him, keeping Hunglu in sight. If he moved out of sight, the bird quickly flew after him.

Darkness had fallen by the time the two of them reached the cabin. Hunglu lit a small oil lamp, mashed some nuts, and fed his bird. He then took a leather bundle from the side of his bed and untied the rawhide cords that bound it. Unwrapping the two layers of leather, a long two-handed, double-edged sword was revealed. The sword had arrived nearly a year after Hunglu came to the monastery. There was a scroll with it that read:

The strongest sword is the sword of the mind.
Let this sword cut through your problems
Until the time we fly again.

It was signed by Li.

The sword was a present to Hunglu. Two years after the mission, Li had come to the monastery to rest while on a journey to the east. He stayed for a month and taught Hunglu the forms of this rare sword.

After today's life review, Hunglu felt a need to cut through the discord of his mind. With the parrot secure and sleeping, he quietly left the cabin. The moon was rising above the valley as Hunglu reached his small training area.

He stood motionless, looking at the waxing moonrise and breathing slowly. Only at night did Hunglu dare to remove his shirt, but when he did, it invigorated him. The cool air felt sublime against his bare skin and there was no coarse material to chafe his old wounds as he practiced his exercises. Sword in hand, he began to move slowly, parrying imaginary cuts and countering with slashes and thrusts. This particular sword pattern started very slowly, like Tai Chi, then continually increased in tempo until the movements were at full combat speed. The exercise required the absolute integration of the body and sword if one wished to remain balanced. The sword was too big to be muscled with the arms; it had to be moved with the entire body. As Hunglu's body moved the sword, the weapon provided him with feedback. Every correct stroke made the sword feel like it was pulling him, and at the end of each movement Hunglu could feel a pulse through both his body and sword. But the most important benefit he received from the sword was the release of anger and tension from his lower energy centers.

Though deep in his past, Hunglu needed to release the tension of his warrior days. He never recovered from seeing the tragic souls of people he killed with the bomb. He wondered, sometimes, had *he* died that day where would his soul have gone?

Hunglu earned himself a legendary status with his heroism, yet he could not atone for the taking of a life in ambush. There was no honor in surprising and impersonally killing people without giving them the opportunity to defend themselves.

Hunglu continued wielding the massive weapon and listening to the slicing sound it made in the air. The sword glinted in the moonlight, firing bright reflections against the trees and Hunglu's cabin. Sweat poured down his flesh, and he felt as if the sword was now pulling not only his body with its great weight but also his mind. Deep in concentration, his hand blending with the base of the sword, Hunglu felt himself moving slightly backward in time.

The moonlight glistened off the blade, he was now moving at a speed that surpassed any he had achieved previously. Hunglu's body was alive, his mind clear, his heart at peace.

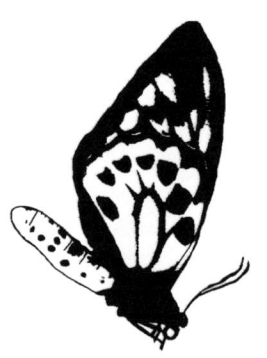

MOON OVER THE WATER

The first time he met the Grandmaster, Moon Over the Water, Hunglu was barely conscious. Shortly after Li, Pi, Hou, and Yin left him at the monastery Hunglu regained consciousness and opened his eyes to Moon Over the Water.

"I know you," Hunglu whispered, his voice hoarse and weak.

"Yes, you do, Flying Spirit," the Grandmaster replied.

The two of them looked at each other for a long time, but neither spoke another word that day.

Moon Over the Water was a master of Yin forces, and taught Hunglu that in Taoist philosophy everything existed within a vast void called Tao. The Tao was so immense and complex that it couldn't be understood from the perspective of a human being. It was, therefore, a Taoist practice to try to understand the workings of the Tao by studying nature. Taoists saw that patterns found in the lowest creatures were duplicated in larger creatures, that the microcosm was a reflection of the *macro*cosm, and that to understand oneself was to know the universe. Within Tao lay the Wu Chi. Wu Chi, Moon Over the Water explained, was the energy of a thought, of an intention. Once the intention started to take form, then Tai Chi began.

It was not easy for Hunglu to grasp these concepts at first, and the Grandmaster had to explain them many times. Sometimes they would spend hours together, Moon Over the Water helping Hunglu to learn the philosophies of the Tao, like a parent teaching a child necessary skills to survive in a vast, confusing world. In many ways, Hunglu had been plucked from the edge of disaster, ferried to the monastery by nothing more than fate, and given a chance to start life anew.

The Grandmaster told Hunglu that Tai Chi was the harmony of the polarities of Yin and Yang. The polarities, though, were not in opposition. Instead, the Yin and Yang existed to define each other, just as light defined dark. The Yin and Yang, in combination, created existence: Yin, the *pervasive* force, was the *medium* of creation, while Yang was the *active* force of creation. Yin would be the canvas and Yang the painting, Moon Over the Water said by way of example. It took many months before Hunglu could even fully comprehend this explanation. The Grandmaster told his pupil to be patient, that most true understanding was not ever accomplished simply with words.

Moon Over the Water was born of privilege, the fifth son of a northern warlord. Not having the temperament for battle, he was moved into civil service as an imperial administrator at the northern capital. He was curious about the Taoist religion and started to spend many hours at the temple, studying with the abbot. After ten years of administration and Taoist study, he felt a calling to learn the mysticism of Taoism. The abbot referred him to a temple in southwestern China, far from the influences of his father and the imperial city.

Enjoying the complexity of the paradoxical philosophy of Taoism, Moon Over the Water found the lush rituals and prayers even more appealing. He studied hard and was ordained as a priest. He loved what he saw as a scientific process of religion, how each aspect of Taoist religion was designed to achieve a specific effect in moving a believer forward in a spiritual process. With over three hundred different sects ranging between monastic and secular practice, Taoism certainly had something to offer everyone who chose to practice it.

What Moon Over the Water discovered was that the mystical process was the foundation of *all* the teachings. Most practitioners tended to be secular, looking for blessings and guidance, but to understand the universe one had to leave physical life behind and explore the Yin side of human existence. Practicing the Yin meant finding harmony and not taking a position in human affairs. Moon Over the Water went to great lengths to learn, practice, and define the esoteric Taoist meditation processes.

His grandmaster had Moon Over the Water specialize in Tai Chi, Chi Kung exercises, and the staff as a weapon. Further, Moon Over the Water's scholarly approach to Taoism, combined with his passion to explore the Yin side of life, qualified him to become a traveling emissary to other lands, sharing what he had learned and exploring new techniques and processes of other monasteries. Moon Over the

Water was being groomed for a special purpose: to be a wandering Taoist. It was a great honor. Wandering Taoists were monks who truly moved with the Tao, going synergistically from location to location, without thought. They followed their intuitions and visions and were always in the right place at the right time. They had no roots, no destination. Their purpose was only to learn and share their knowledge. Wandering Taoists had to live off the land and their wits. Such autonomy required the careful study of plants and herbs for both food and medicinal purposes.

Like a leaf in a stream, the wandering Taoist exercised the Yin principles of passivity and reflection. These principles were how Moon Over the Water received his name. The moon's brightness did not come from itself, it reflected the light of the greater source: the sun. It was this property that made the first part of the monk's name suitable to his personality. The second part also had special significance. Water, reflective but never aggressive, could passively wear away deep canyons and amass itself to destroy whole cities. Water could not itself be destroyed, it could only be altered in form. All the water upon the earth had been there since creation. Water always sought the lowest level and passively adjusted itself to its surroundings. It was essential to all life. Once one rooted himself deeply in the teachings of Taoism, he too was as eternal as water, a part of the never-ending ebb and flow of life.

After twelve years of training, Moon Over the Water started his thirty-year journey to study the world around him. Being from the north, he preferred the cooler climates of the mountains, so he traveled to India and learned the Hindu religion, Buddhism, Hatha Yoga, and Dharma Yoga. Then he traveled north to Tibet and studied Tibetan Buddhism. It was in Tibet that he first met the Butterfly Immortal in a meditation. He was told to go back to China and enter the Gateway of Heaven monastery. During the trip back over the mountains, the Butterfly Immortal walked with Moon Over the Water, taught him, and told him of the future—a future that described the coming of an important monk, a quiet man marked by great scars on his back.

Moon Over the Water had been at the Gateway to Heaven monastery for three years when Hunglu arrived. Upon meeting, Hunglu could tell that this man had a depth of knowledge, metaphysical skill, and life experience that made his words like gold. But Hunglu spent weeks in and out of consciousness before he was ready to grab firmly onto the here-and-now. This dreamlike state provided many adventures and lessons that went uncensored by the conscious mind and ego. His unconscious was reprogramming itself and laying the foundation for the work that would come. Moon Over the Water knew that the immortals were doing their work in Hunglu's mind. He checked in every day and made sure he was there when Hunglu's grasp on reality held. Finally the day came when Hunglu emerged from his wounded haze.

"Welcome back," Moon Over the Water said. "Your wounds are healing well."

"Am I dead?" Hunglu asked.

"No, not yet," the Grandmaster answered. "I am Moon Over the Water, Grandmaster of the Gateway to Heaven monastery. You were brought here three weeks ago by Master Li. You have very serious burns on the back of your body. You have been healing and learning on other planes, and now you are home."

Now you are home.

Those words echoed in Hunglu's mind. It had been so long since he thought of anywhere as home. He instantly felt safe with this man whom he recognized from a dream.

"I saw you when I was with my mother and father, after . . . the accident."

"Yes, that was me," the Grandmaster confirmed.

"But how?" Hunglu asked weakly. "I was dead, and you were . . . *there?* Now you say I am alive and you are *here?*"

"One of the many powers of the mind," the Grandmaster said in a comforting voice. "You too will learn that skill in time. For now we have to heal your body."

"How long will I be here?" Hunglu asked, wondering if he would be forced to leave when he recovered.

"As long as you wish to be a part of our family," the Grandmaster replied.

Family, Hunglu thought. A family was what he wanted most. Then he wondered about his uncle.

"Your uncle has been notified by Master Li," the Grandmaster continued, as if reading Hunglu's mind. "And General Kwan sends his regards. You are a hero. You changed the history of China by your actions."

"I have nothing to be proud of," Hunglu lamented. "What I did had no honor. It was a coward's way."

"Not so. Two men against an army would have been death for you," the Grandmaster countered. "You used the best weapon for the circumstances. In wartime, honorable men often must do dishonorable things to survive. There is no shame in that. Honor, however, is a state of being that you possess when you believe that what you are doing is right and truthful, *at the time you are doing it*. You saved thousands of lives on both sides with your actions, so focus on the good that you accomplished."

"Grandmaster, after the bomb went off I left my body . . . *and* I could see the spirits of the men I killed. I could feel their feelings . . . and their thoughts." Hunglu's voice was low and his eyes shifted around. "Before the bomb went off, I could not think of anything but killing these men for the good of the empire. But when I saw their spirits, I saw them as confused men like myself. I felt sadness and loss . . . and something happened afterward that frightened me."

"What was that?" the Grandmaster asked gently.

"Lord Chu looked at me as if he meant to kill me. But then he realized we were not . . . *real*. He started to fold up into a black box . . . and the box kept getting deeper and darker and harder, and I could *feel* what he felt. I could feel fear and a great emptiness . . . an emptiness to the core of his soul."

"Yes, you watched a man whose material and selfish concerns were greater than his spiritual awareness. You saw a man denounce his spiritual self and heritage to create a self-imposed exile from the light of heaven." The Grandmaster nodded his head, as if he knew from his experiences.

"Is it the Hell the texts talk about?" Hunglu asked.

"No, although it feels like it when you are there." The Grandmaster touched Hunglu's shoulder gently. "And you must stay there until you are willing to believe in the love and light of heaven. But you really aren't alone. You only believe so."

Hunglu was wide-eyed. "Was this because Lord Chu was evil?"

"It has nothing to do with good or evil. It has to do with worshipping the ego," the Grandmaster explained. "Men who choose to live their lives trying to exalt themselves ultimately demean others, overindulge their intellects, and refuse to entertain the belief in a spiritual afterlife—these men have no place to go after they die but into darkness. They create their own little black box by the way they live and what they believe. The stronger the denouncements and intellectual isolation, the deeper and denser the box." The Grandmaster's face was grim.

Hunglu recalled another moment for the Grandmaster. "There was a soldier fighting with invisible enemies over his body. I could feel his terror, too."

"Some people believe that demons are waiting for them after death, either because they deserve it or because it is their destiny," the Grandmaster said in a matter-of-fact tone.

"But *I* didn't see any demons," Hunglu said, concerned that he could possibly have missed something important.

The Grandmaster smiled. "Of course not, the demons were only a creation of the other man's mind and beliefs. They were the products of his fears and transgressions manifested into a form that could provide learning and atonement. But they were also *very* real to him. Hunglu, the demons of the mind are more powerful than any demon spirit could be. They feed upon fear, they grow stronger from it. Some believe that they are fear incarnate. But they are easily defeated through love and forgiveness. All demons can be easily defeated by facing our truths and fears during life. If they are not defeated in life, we must face them after death."

Hunglu nodded and continued. There was so much he needed to tell the Grandmaster. "One man kept trying to get into his body and pick up weapons. He could not see me or any of the other spirits around him . . . there was even a bright being next to him trying to get his attention."

"Ah yes, this is the saddest course of death." The Grandmaster slowly shook his head with pity. "When people are addicted to life, like wine, they cannot give it up easily. They do not believe in any other possibility and their fear of death is so strong that they refuse to acknowledge it, even *after* it occurs. Their will and desire to hold onto life is so great that they become ghosts that aimlessly try to participate in a physical life that ignores them."

"Are they doomed Grandmaster?" Hunglu asked.

"Not at all," the old man replied. "They learn to accept death, and in time they gain awareness of their circumstances. That is when one of the bright beings will come to guide them to a different place. But you don't have to be concerned about these types of death, Hunglu. Remember your experiences, your freedom, and your bliss instead. Death mirrors life in many ways, and if you live a life of isolation, hatred, suspicion, coldly shutting down your heart, then you will attract that kind of death. Listen to me closely: seek out beauty and knowledge and adventure. Show kindness to others, and you will have a kinder death experience."

"Does your religion teach you these things?" Hunglu asked.

"No, this is learned through a mystical process and practicing meditation. Our religion only provides us a context for understanding what we are experiencing and provides rules to keep us safe. Rules, prayers, and rituals, that's what Taoism is all about, Hunglu."

Hunglu frowned at the thought, recalling his childhood efforts to memorize prayers, the names of all the deities and the holy days.

The Grandmaster smiled, as if reading his mind again. "There will come a time in your adventures when all those deities will become real. Then the Taoist religion, along with all other religions, will make sense to you. But for now, you must rest. I will come again tomorrow and we will continue."

The Grandmaster looked at Hunglu sympathetically, then rose to leave.

Hunglu realized he was very tired after the long discussion. As he drifted into a deep sleep, he noticed a feeling of relief begin to wash over his concerns about the killing.

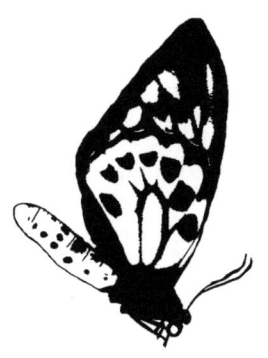

REBIRTH

The Grandmaster reappeared the next day promptly after the morning meal. "Today, you must learn to breathe!" he commanded as he entered the room. There was little time for Hunglu to react before he found himself standing on wobbly legs and taking deep breaths.

The Grandmaster started Hunglu's training with a lesson on reverse breathing, teaching him how to move the tan tein to activate his Chi energy.

In reverse breathing, Hunglu was made to concentrate on the abdominal muscles below his navel. Beneath those muscles was a reservoir of non-physical energy called Chi, the Grandmaster told him. The psychic energy center was called the tan tein. By focusing his mind on the tan tein at the same time he breathed and contracted the lower abdominal muscles, Hunglu activated a flow of Chi energy. He circulated the energy stored in the tan tein by contracting the muscles inward as he inhaled and relaxing the muscles as he exhaled.

"This is awkward," Hunglu complained to his master, but he continued practicing. In a few minutes he had the tempo and coordination in place.

Then the Grandmaster asked Hunglu to imagine a wave of energy moving up the back of his legs to the top of his head as he inhaled. When he exhaled, Hunglu opened his mind and felt a wave moving down the front of his body to his feet.

"Why do I have to do this? I mean, what will it accomplish?" Hunglu asked after few hours.

"Come here." The Grandmaster said. He had been trained in very detailed and intense forms of breath work and energy circulation from a variety of yoga and Chi Kung systems. Through all those years of experience, he learned that the simplest methods worked best with new students. The Grandmaster took Hunglu's hand and placed it on his tan tein. Then the Grandmaster breathed a few cycles and raised a one-inch diameter hemispherical welt. "Follow the movement with your hand," the old man commanded.

Hunglu was surprised to find that the Grandmaster could create a welt and was even more surprised when it moved. The Grandmaster shifted the welt all over his body, first along the Chi meridians, then wherever he wanted.

"This is amazing!" Hunglu exclaimed.

"Not so. It is a trick," the Grandmaster said. "It teaches you how to control the body with the mind when healing. But it has no *real* value. There are many magical tricks that can be learned through discipline and meditation. Each has a purpose to demonstrate that nothing is impossible, and they can provide a goal where the more ambitious students may focus their training. But, Hunglu, we believe in the tenet, *know magic, shun magic*! It is important to have goals and realize for yourself that, through experience, you are an infinitely powerful, immortal being. To know this, you must do things that seem impossible to your beliefs and the society around you. You must eventually defy the laws that govern physical existence. But after you do magic, after you move objects with your mind or other such feats, you must immediately give it up."

"Why?"

"Because," the Grandmaster said sternly, "the powers become like opium, an addiction to illusions that provide escape and ego gain. The drive to obtain power is fueled by weaknesses in our minds. Every power we obtain is a compensation for that weakness. If we hold on to the power, we also retain the weakness. When we let go of the power, then and only then do we release the weakness within us. If you become attached to what you have, you will never see what you could have instead. Remember, there is always another challenge to overcome and a new skill to master. Every soul has a purpose to accomplish goals, which may take *many* lifetimes to achieve. There are challenges which stand in the way of achieving one's purpose. So a soul designs multiple lifetimes to acquire the knowledge and master the skills required to achieve its ultimate purpose. To be in harmony with your soul, you must learn and experience many things. Becoming attached or addicted to any element of your life limits your soul's ability to learn what it needs. The soul will learn what it needs

106

with or without your cooperation. Of course, it is always better to cooperate. Now back to work."

Hunglu practiced breathing and circulating energy waves. He was able to feel a tingling around his body when a wave moved over it. The tingling turned into a deeper sensation that vibrated through his body.

"Grandmaster, is this Chi I'm feeling?"

"Chi is a force that you cannot feel—it is not physical. What you are feeling are the *results* of the Chi, how the Chi affects your body. The intention of your mind directs the Chi to parts of your body and the Chi will follow the path, whether you feel it or not. Sometimes we feel sensations of temperature or tingling that we believe are Chi, but in truth are not. They are created by our posture, body tension, or the movement of our blood. To test the nonphysical nature of a sensation, simply move. Real Chi sensations will continue no matter what posture you are in. It is the mind that matters, not the body."

"So then, the mind is the most important part?" Hunglu asked.

"Exactly, Hunglu," the Grandmaster said. "The intention of the mind, both conscious and unconscious, controls and directs the flow of Chi through the body. If the intention is positive and strong, the flow is good; if the intention is negative and unfocused, the flow will be weakened. Now, let's continue our exercises. The bones are a source of strength and power, so imagine the bones glowing and lighting up as they fill with universal Chi energy. Imagine that light glowing outward in all directions. . ."

Hunglu could feel his bones begin to light up and radiate outward into his body. It felt warm and energizing. He could feel the pain of the burns dissolving and his body disappearing into the light.

After his initial guided instruction, Hunglu practiced his exercises every day. The results were excellent and the burns healed far quicker than he imagined.

As he became stronger, the Grandmaster taught him Chi Kung exercises to stimulate the Chi flow through the body.

Chi Kung exercises were a part of the medical arts. There were many different types and sets of Chi Kung, but they all relaxed the body, improved the circulation of Chi, realigned the structures of the body, and stretched and conditioned the body. Chi Kung combined breathing with repetitive movements—up to a thousand repetitions of the same movement—which opened blockages of Chi and the mind. The repetitive motion moved the practitioner into a deep meditative state for a long period of time, causing disrupted and chaotic thinking processes to erode.

The first Chi Kung exercises Hunglu learned were regenerative, specifically designed to heal wounds and build physical strength. He then learned a series of Chi Kung exercises that balanced the energy centers of the body and improved the overall condition. These exercises were generally used to prevent illness. Hunglu practiced them daily to regain balance. Only when he became stronger did the Grandmaster attempt to teach him Tai Chi Chuan.

"This will help to set you free," Moon Over the Water told Hunglu.

In Tai Chi Chuan, Hunglu found an art that combined the healing practices of Chi Kung with martial-arts applications. Unlike Chi Kung, Tai Chi movements continually changed from one posture and form to another. The ever-changing nature of Tai Chi was believed to be reflective of the ever-changing nature of the Tao itself, the Grandmaster said.

Hunglu discovered that the repetitive nature of Chi Kung induced meditative states, but the more complex forms of Tai Chi challenged those states. Chi Kung exercises were performed from side to side, exchanging one movement for its mirror image, repeating both throughout the practice. Tai Chi form was a dance of different movements performed in a sequence.

As the Grandmaster instructed his student, Hunglu sometimes remembered his experiences with his bodyguard, Lu, from years before. Though Lu had taught Hunglu the Tiger style of fighting, Lu also practiced Tai Chi.

"I can't believe you can defend yourself with those slow movements!" Hunglu taunted Lu.

"Then try to hit me, young one," Lu suggested.

Hunglu launched a brazen flurry of punches but ended up on the ground, quite unsure of how he got there.

"How do you do that?" Hunglu exclaimed as Lu laughed.

"I don't do much of *anything*." Lu smiled at Hunglu's bewilderment. "You provided the force, I just assumed one of the postures and danced with you until you fell."

The Grandmaster, years later, taught Hunglu a similar lesson: "You must never use any force, you must be completely Yin, like water. Always let the opponent enter into you. This requires fearlessness to succeed. The Tai Chi master possesses the fearlessness to stand in the face of a charging tiger and not move until the claws are just a hair's breadth away."

Hunglu sat still, admiring the Grandmaster's boldness.

"A tiger would never charge a Tai Chi master," Moon Over the Water said.

"Why not?" Hunglu asked.

"A Tai Chi master takes no position—he neither contends nor competes. And because he does not contend, he is in harmony with all things and will not be attacked. Now, let's continue."

"Keep your body absolutely relaxed, with no tension at all, so that you can wrap around your opponent like a snake coils around its prey. Be supple and smooth in your movements. Be like water, offering no resistance and enveloping that which presses upon you, drowning it with your being, not with your body."

Hunglu's blank expression clearly showed his lack of understanding of this concept.

The Grandmaster knew better than to force this skill onto Hunglu at such an early stage. "Someday, you'll experience it and then you will understand," he chuckled. "For now, you must have no plan or expectation of what technique to use. The direction of the forces that the opponent applies to you will push you into the proper technique. Just remember that this requires a calm, tranquil mind that flows with whatever is presented."

The Grandmaster had Hunglu close his eyes and place his hands palm to palm with the Grandmaster's. Then the Grandmaster moved his hands and asked Hunglu to follow without losing contact.

The exercise was very difficult until Hunglu learned to relax. As he calmed, he felt his hands becoming very soft against the Grandmaster's hands. He could even feel the pulse and blood beneath his own skin. Before he relaxed, Hunglu did not even feel the Grandmaster's hands, but as he became more serene the old man's hands felt solid and were easy to follow.

The Grandmaster started to move all around the courtyard, changing levels and even using blocking techniques to strip Hunglu's hands from him. For hours on end the teacher and the student could be seen moving about in a graceful dance, locked together by nothing more than will—a most powerful bond, Hunglu discovered. Only when Hunglu could follow the Grandmaster around the courtyard without losing contact did the Grandmaster increase the training regiment.

"You have learned to follow your partner's body and intentions," the Grandmaster began one morning in the courtyard. "Now you must learn to move to the partner's center to control the action. To do this you follow the contours of the partner's arms to the center of the body. Your hands must slither up an arm like a snake up a tree, silently, smoothly, without detection. The hands must traverse the arms and find the head or chest."

The Grandmaster showed Hunglu how to follow a partner's action and then, with a simple twisting contour, how to take a position behind the partner, neutralizing the action. Hunglu's first attempt at the maneuver was eager but unskilled. It lacked any grace at all.

"Hunglu, you must *not* practice Tai Chi as a martial art if you wish to achieve its benefits," the Grandmaster admonished. "Otherwise you will find yourself focusing on the applications of the technique rather than understanding the movement at its deepest energy level. I will teach you the movements, but *do not* try to understand the applications. You must trust that your body and spirit know how to use them at the appropriate time."

The Grandmaster taught Hunglu a posture movement that would have thrown a lesser man off balance. His body moved back and forth rhythmically, like a willow being blown in the wind. Hunglu was directed to repeat the movement and its mirror in this manner hundreds of times. Finally, the moves became smooth and were inextricably burned into his mind, while the steady side-to-side motion sent Hunglu into a meditative trance.

"You must try to have the same state of mind here that you have when you travel outside your body," the Grandmaster instructed. "But also feel your feet firmly upon the ground. Feel the body completely and let the mind and spirit expand as far as they will go."

When Hunglu had achieved the fluidity of mind, body, and spirit for several different posture movements, the Grandmaster taught him how everything fit together into a form set of individual moves. "The challenge is to continue the sensations of the side-to-side motions from the sequence of one move into the next."

Though Hunglu began to experience the freedom the Grandmaster had spoken of, he was also beginning to feel restricted again as the lessons continued.

"Why do we repeat the same sequence and not use a more spontaneous series?" he asked during one session.

"There are many reasons for this," the Grandmaster began. "The first is that spontaneous movement will lead you only to the movements that you like and can do the best. Important movements that you *need* to know and those movements that you are weak in will not develop. The second reason is that you must develop a spontaneous expression within the structure of the sequence. Then you can discover freedom within the form. You have a body which has limits, yet your mind has learned to travel outside your body, allowing you to locate freedom within *your* form."

Hunglu smiled, as he clearly understood the example.

"The third and most important reason is to master the patterns of your mind," the Grandmaster continued. "The more you repeat the same pattern over and over, the deeper your understanding of the pattern becomes. You will start to become aware of even more subtle patterns inside and outside your body, and this develops your ability to perceive and understand the patterns of the world around you. These, Hunglu, are the patterns of your mind."

"From now on, you will see more erroneous patterns of life around you. You will be able to predict people's actions and words from the most subtle of clues. As you progress, you will rid your life of all habits and thoughts that are not productive. This is the deepest work of Tai Chi, and Tai Chi Chuan is an art that you will master." The Grandmaster's voice was forceful. "Know this: if one hundred people practice Tai Chi, everyone will receive health and mental benefits. Out of the one hundred, twenty will become technical *experts* of the art. Out of that twenty, ten will become technical *masters* of the art. Out of the ten, only three will master the deepest meanings and metaphysics of the art. Hunglu, you are already one of the three, and now you must rise to your full potential."

Feeling that mantle of responsibility, Hunglu practiced three times a day for three years to achieve technical mastery of his form. During that time, he grew in strength and confidence and spirituality. But it was also during this time that Hunglu focused more on his skills than those around him. He had pleasant but superficial relationships with his fellow monks and had not yet transcended his shyness. It was Hunglu's hope that no one really noticed his awkward nature in large gatherings. He was much better one on one. Like so many people, he just wanted to disappear into the mix. There it was safe and he would have gladly embraced anonymity forever, but fate had other things in store for Hunglu.

TAN

It was common for outside martial artists to come to the monastery and challenge the monks to a test of fighting prowess. The monks practiced many forms of martial arts in their physical and spiritual development. Their great skill was gained by the integration of meditation into their practice, allowing them to access the deepest metaphysical powers of the art.

In fighting, the monks' focus was complete. They were not limited by ego or fear, thus their techniques channeled their inner power into a target. Most of the time the Grandmaster would not participate, but on rare occasions some of the monks were allowed to fight to get necessary experience.

On an autumn day, a thirty-two-year-old fighter named Tan arrived at the temple. Tan, who was also known as the Tiger, was a professional fighter who practiced the southern Five Animal system of fighting. Created at the Shaolin Temple, the Five Animal system consisted of movements that imitated the fighting techniques and spirit of the tiger, panther, snake, crane, and dragon. It was a powerful system that could take a student through different phases of development, ranging from the purely physical use of force to the use of internal Chi techniques.

Tan had been trained by a friend of the Grandmaster, so courtesy dictated he be given an audience. Tan's master was a man who believed in perfection and power. He developed his students through hard work and repetition, spending hours toughening their bodies and techniques by having the students pound trees and stones. Tan's muscular body and perfect forms were a living monument proclaiming his master's success.

Shortly after his arrival, the Grandmaster and Tan called on Hunglu.

"Hunglu, Tan has consented to help with your understanding of Tai Chi principles," the Grandmaster said. "However, you must

113

follow some rules. You must not use your feet, you must not strike, you must only contour against your opponent's attacks. Tan, on the other hand, may do anything he wants."

Hunglu, though surprised and confused, trusted his grandmaster and accepted the challenge with a humble nod.

In the center of the courtyard, Hunglu stood with bent knees and lifted his arms as if he was going to practice with the Grandmaster. Tan circled and stalked, sure that the fight would be over shortly. Hunglu calmed himself, as if he was holding the ball in the forest.

Suddenly, Tan moved forward and dropped to one knee, swinging the other leg hard into Hunglu's calves, but to Tan's surprise his strike bounced off Hunglu. Tan quickly recovered but Hunglu had not felt a thing.

Tan feigned a few strikes, then launched a full-powered Tiger-claw strike to Hunglu's head. To Hunglu it was like Tan was moving in slow motion. Just before the strike made contact, Hunglu lifted his left hand and slid it up Tan's forearm, redirecting the claw above his head. The movement made Tan fall slightly forward into Hunglu's elbow. There was a soft *thud* as he bounced off Hunglu and fell to the ground.

"What did you *do!*" Tan shouted at Hunglu.

"I don't know," Hunglu responded truthfully.

The Grandmaster laughed at both of them, "That's enough! You have both done very well."

The Grandmaster called them into his quarters. Over tea, he explained the martial theory of Tai Chi Chuan. It was from that day on that Hunglu never doubted the defensive ability of Tai Chi, nor did he ever practice the art with martial intention again. It remained locked within him, a secret knowledge known only to masters.

THE RULER

Hunglu floated over white-capped mountains and beyond the sky. Finding a shimmering temple, he was drawn through a pair of thin crystalline doors and entered a vast room lit with hundreds of candles reflecting off the walls. Within the shrine there was an intricately carved gold relief depicting the story of the gods and creation, and on a platform before the shrine sat the Butterfly Immortal himself. Though pulsing with brilliant light, Hunglu could see his master clearly. The immortal had a kind, wise face, and he had opened his arms in an inviting gesture.

"Welcome, Flying Spirit, we have much to discuss tonight," the Butterfly Immortal said. "The progress on your self-review is going very well, but we still have some other levels of life to explore. Take your position, and we will begin." Hunglu lowered to his knees and listened intently as the immortal began to lecture him.

"Human life, Hunglu, is a combination of the mind and body and spirit coordinating their efforts to assist the soul in accomplishing its life mission. But all this must be done in harmony with the universe to achieve the higher purposes of the Tao. Nothing works alone. For example, the bark, wood, and sap of a tree all work together for the growth of the tree, yet the tree is a part of the larger earth. It *needs* the life forces that the ground supplies. It *needs* the light and rain from the sky. The tree's leaves then become food for insects and other plants, and its fruits and seeds feed the birds and animals. Just as the tree is important to the larger earth, each life is important to the earth and the Tao in ways you cannot yet imagine.

"How you function from this point on depends upon the relationship between your mind, body, and spirit, Hunglu. If they work in harmony, you are living a life of virtue and can achieve immortality. The body is the medium through which a life expresses itself in reality; its movements form expressions, which can be read.

The body is also a storage box for Chi energy, which it can share with the earth around it. But if a life focuses *too much* on the body, expression is limited."

"You have seen martial artists who have spent all their lives working on skills. They become excellent technical masters of their art, but they don't know the classics or believe much in the power of the spirit. Their singular focus upon the physical prevents them from having an experience like you are having now. The spirit is the power of life. It comes from the soul, and the soul is a living piece of the universal god. Harmonizing with the soul allows access to the core power of all things, providing universal knowledge of everything that is, will be, or ever has been."

The new ideas the Butterfly Immortal expressed were confusing to Hunglu. In his studies of Taoism he had learned about many deities, and through meditation and ritual he had come to believe in the existence and power of these deities. However, Hunglu never really grasped the concept of a universal god like the Butterfly Immortal was talking about.

The Butterfly Immortal saw the confusion on his student's face and continued carefully. "The mind is created by the body and the soul. The Yang, or active mind, is created by the people and events around you: teachers, parents, government, and experiences, whether good or bad. The Yang mind determines how you will interact within your world. It processes your beliefs and fears and develops appropriate actions and words. The Yin mind, on the other hand, is created by your soul. It is your basic nature and determines the underlying imperative for your lifetime. The Yang mind provides the human skills, knowledge, and limitations; the Yin mind provides the *imperative direction* in which to use these talents. Together they guide a life to complete its purpose.

"But you should know, Hunglu, that most minds limit the functions of their soul. These limits often come from a person's upbringing and their beliefs. Such limits can prevent men from doing what their souls desire. Then resistance causes unhappiness and disease, until finally, the soul will force the life and the lives around it to give it the lessons it needs. This is a difficult process for all involved. There is much sadness and struggle."

"Master, what does the soul need from us?" Hunglu asked.

"The soul is like a baby," the Butterfly Immortal answered. "It learns through experience. Each experience forges, strengthens, and shapes the soul. Like a child, the more a soul learns, the more powerful and interactive it becomes. As the soul obtains more perspective, its lessons change to gather different experiences. This will help it to be more effective in its imperative."

"Master, what is this *imperative?*" Hunglu prodded, curious about the idea.

"Do not be concerned if you are at first confused—be patient and ask questions as I explain. Mostly, though, open your mind. The ideas will settle in time.

"There are eight imperatives used to describe souls. There is also an imperative lesson that needs to be learned by each soul in a lifetime. The imperative class defines the objectives and role of the soul from the perspective of the Tao, determining which deities govern it. An imperative lesson is the particular motivation for the soul's current life experience. The imperative lesson directs how the life should work and helps one make decisions in order to learn that lesson. The lessons are learned in a sequence: the Security Imperative, the Power Imperative, the Freedom Imperative, the Love Imperative, the Justice Imperative, the Progressive Imperative, the Humanitarian Imperative, and the Universal Imperative. Each lesson is expressed differently, according to the type of soul classification it has.

"The Security Imperative soul will always be working for the survival and preservation of itself and those around it. It will base all of its decisions on the belief that it is providing support and safety for itself, family, clan, and society. A Security Imperative soul living a security-imperative lifetime may be a homeless peasant dealing with survival without any skills to better his situation. A Security Imperative soul in a power lifetime may be a thief. In a freedom lifetime, it may be a nomadic herder. The Security Imperative is like the skin on your body: large and absolutely vital for your survival."

"The Power Imperative is also concerned with survival, but its primary focus is on individual power and control over its surroundings. It wishes to attain recognition, to become a leader in its society. It manipulates ideas, objects, and finances for the good of both the society and itself."

"The Freedom Imperative is concerned with removing oppression by disrupting the control of the Power Imperative and challenging the harmony of the Security Imperative. The Freedom Imperative exists primarily to balance power and security."

"The Love Imperative bonds and connects to other souls. It is the path of finding beauty and grace within the workings of the mind. It can become a chameleon, blending with whomever it is with. The Love Imperative spreads joy."

"The Justice Imperative is the master of will and intention. It creates order among the souls. But it is not inclined to become a social leader, as the Power Imperative is. It measures its effectiveness by the amount of fairness and equality it can create."

"The Progressive Imperative creates evolution in society and technology. It was a progressive who invented the wheel, Hunglu. A soul with the Progressive Imperative lives only to produce innovation, without any concern for the self."

"The Humanitarian Imperative exists to serve its fellow humans. It has no purpose or meaning outside of promoting the health and harmony of those around it. The Humanitarian Imperative is invisible, its works are hidden, it shuns all recognition for its wondrous deeds."

"At last, there is the Universal Imperative, which rarely takes human form. It exists to connect and harmonize the workings of souls with the Yin nature of the Tao." And there the Butterfly Immortal ended, his glow dimming almost imperceptibly.

Hunglu took in all his master told him, but some things he asked the teacher to repeat. The Butterfly Immortal was patient, guiding Hunglu to see the immense value in understanding the imperatives.

Strangely, Hunglu found that most of the imperatives described qualities within him. He remembered events from his life that seemed to point to the surfacing of one imperative or another. At the same time, *none* of the imperatives seemed to apply to him because he did not fit their definition exactly. Security, power, freedom, love, justice, progress, and humanitarianism: these were all things that he strove for at one time or another, but they were all ideas that he had never fully embraced. Throughout life, Hunglu shifted from one imperative to the next as different imperatives met the needs of a situation he found himself in. Didn't everyone do this he wondered? Wasn't it necessary? Hunglu posed the conundrum to his teacher.

"A soul will always retain its imperative class, but it will also change its imperative lesson from life to life," the Immortal explained. "Each life passes through imperatives, but as stages within a lesson. So a security-imperative soul living a power-imperative life will have a humanitarian stage *within* that lifetime. It is perfectly normal and desirable, Hunglu."

"The constant growth, evolution, and flow of imperatives was the inspiration for the *I Ching*, the *Book of Changes*. The *I Ching* is a means to determine the strength and quality of imperative influences at any given time in a life. It was created as a tool for the common people who have not yet learned to access their souls to obtain meaningful guidance and direction. That is why all people must do a life review—to find the true self underneath the Yang mind."

Hunglu eagerly spoke up, "How does one become immortal?"

"Death comes from a weak Yang mind that cannot accept that it is a spirit body in a dream," the Immortal answered. "All souls are immortal, but a soul that has progressed through many lessons—an old soul—develops its own intelligence and expression. The soul controls its imperative and designs *many* lifetimes that will harmonize the Yang mind with the Yin mind. In the end, there is the creation of a *soul being* that can move through spiritual and physical dimensions at will. A soul being realizes life is a dream, and it walks from dream to dream without changing form."

The Butterfly Immortal looked at Hunglu, who had the face of a child now—expectant, ambitious, yearning to learn more. He asked Hunglu if he was ready to begin. Hunglu bowed his head.

"The life review is the first step to cleansing the Yang mind of its limitations. The next step is to completely integrate the mind, body, and spirit. You have spent seven years using Tai Chi Chuan and Chi Kung to fuse your separate parts, now you are ready for another tool. Come forward."

Hunglu stood up and moved toward the master.

The Butterfly Immortal was holding a stick that slowly floated out of his hand and into the air in front of Hunglu's eyes. Hunglu could see that it wasn't an ordinary stick, but a beautifully carved length of reddish-brown wood. Both ends were rounded like half-balls. The carving was about twelve inches in length and about two inches in diameter. The inner section between the balls was much thinner, and in the center of the piece there was a near-perfect sphere. Hunglu could not take his eyes off it. It was as if the tiny spheroid had an aperture that opened and closed, releasing waves of serenity. Hunglu felt intoxicated with its energy, and he was consumed by the power of his gift; all else seemed to disappear.

Sometime later, when Hunglu finally took his mind from the sphere, he found himself lying in his bed. He looked up and saw the carving floating over his head. In his mind, Hunglu heard the Butterfly Immortal's last words: *This is the Tai Chi ruler. It will help you harmonize the Yang of the physical world with the Yin of the spirit world. This is my gift to you.*

Hunglu reached out and grabbed the ruler, which was still floating in the air above him. It was truly an incredible gift.

CHANG TZU

Hunglu woke to the sound of the parrot squawking in his left ear.

"Good morning to you too, little one," he said.

The parrot was now able to forage for most of its food. Though it still needed supplemental feedings, it was becoming very independent. In the past two weeks the parrot had decided to call to Hunglu whenever he started drifting too far into daydreams or other mental distractions. At first Hunglu was upset with the interruptions, but he soon realized the parrot was helping him stay in reality. Hunglu also notice that the parrot only interrupted him during unfocused lapses; it did not interrupt Hunglu in his meditations. It was because of the parrot that Hunglu was taking more notice of his natural surroundings.

"The Grandmaster is right again, little one," Hunglu said. "Before you arrived I was escaping from life, not paying any attention to the reality around me."

Stepping out of the cabin, the sky was gently lit with the rising sun. Hunglu felt cool dew under his feet and a breeze washed the last of his sleep away. He chose a light but invigorating exercise to start the day. The sun continued to grow stronger, brightening the milky clouds hanging over the mountains.

After his Tai Chi practice, Hunglu retrieved his Tai Chi ruler and called out to the bird: "Come, little one! It's time to visit the Grandmaster."

It had been two weeks since Hunglu last talked to the Grandmaster, who had left Hunglu alone to learn from the Butterfly Immortal. Now as Hunglu walked the path to the compound, he was more aware of every footstep and smell than he had ever been in the past. The parrot flew short jaunts from tree to tree as he walked. Although able to fly, the parrot's landings were still comical and this made Hunglu laugh more than once as he watched the parrot consistently miss the branch it was aiming for, then tumble onto another.

"Good thing you parrots have hard heads!" Hunglu called out.

Squawk ack-rohooot! the bird shot back, making Hunglu laugh even more.

Hunglu realized that reflecting on his past lightened his mind and attitude. He also realized he was talking a lot more to the bird.

Moon Over the Water was expecting Hunglu and met the young monk as he walked up the path.

"Hello, Flying Spirit, come with me," the Grandmaster said immediately.

Hunglu smiled and joined Moon Over the Water for a walk up the mountain. Although an old man by normal standards, the Grandmaster had not yet reached his physical peak, and Hunglu had to work to maintain his pace. Moon Over the Water's energy was not surprising; it was he who had walked across the Himalayan mountains years before when he was on his own spiritual quest.

The two men hiked up to a high overlook that the Grandmaster had made into a sacred meditation grotto. There was a small stream that flowed from the top of the mountain and created a little waterfall that fell into a reflecting pool. Together, they drank from the pool. The water was sweet and filled with powerful energy. Then they rested on a bench.

The parrot, which had long ago took refuge on Hunglu's shoulder, now hopped off to explore the grotto floor. It found a cherry branch and occupied itself by chewing the rubbery bark while the two men talked.

"I understand that you received a new gift," the Grandmaster said as he removed his own ruler from his robe.

"Is there anything you *don't* know?" Hunglu asked.

The Grandmaster thought for a moment, looked rather seriously at Hunglu, then said, "No."

"What do I do with this Master? I know it's a tool, but I don't know what it is used for."

The Grandmaster held up his ruler. "This," he said, "will teach you new dimensions of focus and energy projection. Take the ruler and hold it with the rounded ends in both palms. . . now look at the center of the ball and turn it until the grain's eye is facing you.

Hold the ruler in front of you and focus on the eye, Hunglu. Allow your eyes to see what is behind the ball. Keep your focus upon the ball and notice what happens."

Hunglu watched the reddish-brown eye in the center of the ball. In less than a minute his muscles relaxed. Slowly his body started to disappear, but at the same time his peripheral vision increased. He could almost see what was happening behind him. He could feel his heartbeat being transferred into the ruler's ball. There was a pulsing from one palm to the other, and the ruler started to become lighter and lighter until it felt as though it would float away. Suddenly, Hunglu dropped the fantastic instrument.

The bird jumped and the Grandmaster laughed. "You'll drop it many more times" he remarked knowingly. "That is part of the training process."

It took Hunglu a few moments to recover from his deep state of focus as the Grandmaster spoke.

"Your skill will improve so that you don't drop the ruler when you move into deeper states of focused meditation. Part of the goal is to be focused in this reality and other realities at the same time."

Hunglu nodded, understanding what the master meant at a surface level.

"The other part," the Grandmaster added, "is to master the material world, to focus and control objects, including the minds and bodies of others."

Hunglu looked quizzically at the Grandmaster.

"Watch . . ." The Grandmaster leveled his gaze upon Hunglu's ruler, which was still lying on the ground. The ruler floated up into the air and then dropped gently into Hunglu's hands.

"How did you do that?" The words stumbled off Hunglu's tongue as his mind finally began to engage.

"*Practice*," Moon Over the Water said. "Now let's begin again."

The Grandmaster showed Hunglu a sitting meditation posture that used the ruler as a focal point. This required teaching Hunglu how to breathe in a way that directed energy waves through the ruler, not the body. Then the Grandmaster taught him to stand in the Holding-the-Ball position, only with the ruler. The ruler provided a connection between Hunglu's hands and increased the depth of his meditation.

"Why is my focus better when I use the ruler?" Hunglu asked. "It feels deeper, yet I am still here."

"That's a good observation," the Grandmaster said delightedly. "Most meditation is done with the mind and the spirit detached from the body. But the ruler allows you to separate from the Yang aspect of reality and explore the Yin. The ruler helps connect the body to the mind and the spirit, creating an integrated meditation state that is truly a union of the Yin and Yang of life."

"Then this process is more powerful?" Hunglu asked.

"Of course." The Grandmaster smiled at the obvious conclusion. "Otherwise we are just living half a life, achieving only half of our potential."

Hunglu began to wonder what a full-potential life would be like.

"Now we must teach you how to move," the Grandmaster said. "You will use the ruler in the exercise of *Push*."

Hunglu started from a bow-and-arrow stance, his knees bent and one foot placed forward. He shifted his weight back upon the rear leg, pulling the ruler up to eye level, then inhaled to bring energy up to his head. He carefully shifted his weight forward as the body pushed the ruler out and down. Exhaling, the energy flowed down his body.

After Hunglu grew comfortable with the movements, the Grandmaster instructed him to do this a thousand times each day for three years.

"You can begin by spending the next three days here meditating and practicing with the ruler. This will build a good foundation in a natural environment."

Hunglu agreed, looking forward to using the new tool.

The three had their midday meal together, the parrot picking from both the Grandmaster's and Hunglu's bowls. Shortly after, the Grandmaster left, smiling at the prospect of his student's future.

There was enough natural food available for the bird and plenty of water for both of them in the Grandmaster's training ground. Intrigued with the ruler, Hunglu immediately began doing his thousand movements. He found that once his body relaxed, everything moved in complete harmony, smoother than Tai Chi or sword work had been (although he did find the movements similar). In meditation, Hunglu concentrated on how the Grandmaster had levitated the ruler. He knew the Grandmaster was capable of such feats, but this was the first time he had seen one demonstrated so dramatically. Without a doubt, Hunglu knew this was the next level of skill he must achieve.

As he sat, he saw a butterfly float by and was reminded of Chang Tzu's dream and what the Butterfly Immortal had said about the soul.

Chang Tzu drifted away from his normal world into darkness. He felt himself floating in the wind, from the darkness into the sunlight of the dawn. The sun warmed his wings as he flew from flower to flower, dipping his long tongue into the nectar-sweetened dew. His body pulsated with nourishment. He floated upward on a thermal draft, rising above the trees to view mountains bursting with morning mist. From his vista, Chang Tzu was happy with all he experienced. Wind, flight, and nectar were his life. The sun began to set as Chang Tzu folded his wings upon his perch, and he drifted into the darkness of sleep.

In the morning, Chang Tzu woke up with the warmth of the sun upon his face. He rubbed his eyes and rose from his bed among the boughs of the forest. Chang Tzu looked into a clearing filled with wild honeysuckle. Rising to his feet, he walked to the flowers. And as he walked, Chang Tzu suddenly knew he could fly. He remembered the dream of being a butterfly. He knew the taste of nectar and the feel of the wind.

Chang Tzu wondered, 'Am I a man who dreamed I was a butterfly, or am I a butterfly dreaming I am a man?'

Hunglu concluded at that moment that Chang Tzu was both. From his most recent experiences, the monk was beginning to see that the barrier between dream and reality was very thin. He remembered dreams in which he could change events for a more desirable result. He vaguely recalled a dream in which he was running through a forest and slipped on some wet ground. He dropped into the mud, ruining his robe, but deciding that he did not like the outcome, Hunglu repeated his dream without the fall. Now he knew that this was how the Grandmaster moved the ruler—like it was a dream.

Hunglu spent the next day practicing his exercises and meditations, becoming aware that the clarity of his meditations was improving. On the second night, he dreamed of unexpected things.

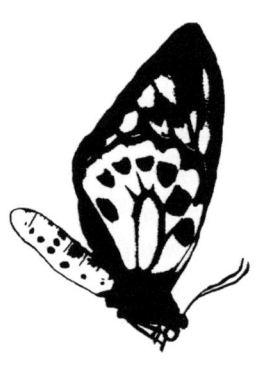

THE DREAM

There were rumors that the princess would be attacked. As part of the escort team, Hunglu was directly responsible for her safety and stayed close by her side. Night was approaching, and the travelers took refuge in a very large cave already occupied by many others. Within the stone walls was a safe haven from the elements. Some of the temporary inhabitants were trustworthy soldiers, and feeling well-supported for the night, Hunglu relaxed.

"We must leave before daybreak to insure her safety," the group leader informed Hunglu before they slept. The three of them rested and prepared for the continuation of their journey.

At dawn the companions exited the cave, wearing hooded robes. Unexpectedly, a man who had been loitering around the mouth of the cave tried to grab the princess. In a flash, Hunglu pulled a dagger from his robe and sliced the man's wrist before the attacker could grab her. He felt the knife cut down to the bone with a sickening scrape. The would-be attacker dropped to his knees in pain.

The princess moved from behind her protectors, knelt down, and held the attacker's wrist with great empathy. She closed her eyes and whispered to him quietly.

Hunglu saw the wound heal before his eyes; the blood flow ceased and the gash closed as if it was being erased.

When the princess stood up, she smiled at Hunglu. "Thank you," she said gently, "but I don't need your defense."

"It is my duty," Hunglu responded even though he could see the princess was a woman of extraordinary powers.

"Will you walk with me?" she asked.

Hunglu followed, stunned by her beauty and the external expression of her inner peace.

"We only need defense if we fear death," the princess said. "We only fear death if we believe we have no control over life. I have an immortal

soul that will live through eternity. If it were my destiny to be killed for that man's learning or some other purpose, there would be no loss. My soul would continue its evolution without disruption. I want to tell you a story, Hunglu.

"Once the Yellow Emperor was given a vicious tiger as a gift. The tiger was roaring and slashing in the cage. General Khan said, 'I can tame that beast for you.' He walked into the cage and beat the tiger over the head with his fan, causing the tiger to cower in the cage. A monk who was also present said, 'That's not the way to do it.' The monk went fearlessly into the cage where the tiger roared furiously. The monk spat upon his hands and walked over to the beast and started petting it. The tiger became very docile and began to purr and rub itself over the monk."

"As you see, Hunglu, the general guaranteed his safety by forcing the beast into submission. He gained control over the tiger only through fear and intimidation. The monk was willing to die to make friends, and in the end he gained a powerful ally."

"If you have nothing to lose, or nothing to defend, you become powerful. This is what Lao Tzu means when he says, 'The man who is in harmony with the Tao has nothing to fear, for there is no place for a rhino to place its horn, or a tiger to place its claw . . .'"

Hunglu woke with a smile upon his face. He was intrigued by his dream because the woman touched his heart in a way he had not felt before. She reached him with a message that made him feel peaceful. With all the skill that Moon Over the Water possessed, and throughout the lands he traveled, he never had to fight with man nor beast. Like the princess, the Grandmaster had a radiant inner peace that made one feel loved.

It would be difficult to attack someone who gave unconditional love, Hunglu concluded. But to love unconditionally required more fearlessness than to do battle.

Hunglu washed his face and started his morning exercises. He began with seated meditation and then moved to standing meditation with the ruler. He did the thousand repetitions of the push drill twice a day. Meanwhile, the parrot practiced its flying, traveling back and forth over the grotto as the other birds were filling the air with song. It was a beautiful morning.

Suddenly, there was silence. In his peripheral vision, Hunglu saw the blue parrot rise into the sky, but with his non-physical eyes he saw a hawk dropping down behind the parrot.

"*No!*" Hunglu shouted as he turned and looked upward. He found himself focusing upon the hawk to the exclusion of everything else. His heart was pounding and there was a terrible fiery sensation spreading across his back—the flesh itself seemed as if it was boiling. The fear of losing his bird overwhelmed Hunglu, yet, in an instant, the fear faded to peace and his consciousness left him. There was an explosion of brown feathers above the parrot, and the hawk fell to the ground, landing ten feet in front of Hunglu. It was destroyed, its neck and wings snapped.

Hunglu held his hand up and the parrot flew to it. He snuggled and petted the blue bird, which was shaking violently from fear. Tears of sadness emptied themselves from Hunglu's heart, making him feel lighter with every drop.

"I almost lost you, little one," he said softly. "I guess I'm not good enough to learn that last lesson."

Hunglu looked at the dead hawk. His mind tried to find another reason for the beast's death, but he knew it was *his* responsibility. He could not even take pride in such a vivid demonstration of his mental powers; the act was not one to celebrate for the man who cherished birds. Instead, he collected the remains of the hawk and placed them in a pile. Then he wept for a long time over the victim.

Late in the afternoon, the Grandmaster appeared.

Hunglu felt like a child in front of his teacher as the Grandmaster attempted to console him.

"What is wrong?"

Hunglu nodded to the hawk. "I killed it," he admitted. "With my thoughts, I ripped it from the sky."

"Oh."

The Grandmaster quickly grasped the gravity of the situation. Hunglu had broken through the reality barrier that demanded all physical things remain separate. He accomplished this feat well before he was prepared to understand the nature of the power and its control. Moon Over the Water knew that the next few moments would be delicate. He met many people who dreamt of having magical powers, but they didn't anticipate the traumatic emotional effects that occurred after their reality crashed. The Grandmaster had seen students crack at this level, then turn to opium rather than further training. However, it was also clear to the Grandmaster that Hunglu had a tremendous emotional breakthrough.

"Tell me what happened," Moon Over the Water said softly.

Hunglu told him the story of the hawk attack and his dream of the previous night. He told the Grandmaster of his fear and emotions when the bird was being attacked and how he wept afterward in both relief and pain.

"Good, good, Flying Spirit, you have had two breakthroughs at the same time," the Grandmaster said. "You have dissolved the limitations of physical reality and experienced an open heart. All your efforts reflecting upon your life have at last allowed you to stop suppressing your emotions, especially love."

"But Grandmaster, all I felt was sadness," Hunglu lamented.

"Sadness is another expression of love, the Yin expression. Sadness and love open the heart to the feeling of union. Love is bonding, it is connecting to another being at a very deep personal level. When a loved one dies, we feel a sadness within us—that is an energy connection to the other person. This sadness is equal to the sensation of bliss. They are the same energy and feeling, but the context is different. We make the mistake of believing bliss will last forever, erroneously anticipating a future with the source of our bliss. In mourning we grieve the lack of a physical future with what we have come to love."

Moon Over the Water watched Hunglu becoming more pensive.

"The connection and feeling between loving beings exists forever." The Grandmaster paused for a moment to stroke Hunglu's hair. "Remember the joy and bliss you felt in the light of death?"

"Yes," Hunglu answered, remembering his childhood experience of nearly drowning in the village well. Again, the image surfaced in his time of need.

"That moment made you shed tears of joy *and* sadness, did it not?" the Grandmaster asked.

"It did," Hunglu answered, now better understanding the Grandmaster when he said there was very little difference between joy and sadness. As Hunglu reflected on his life, he recalled that many times love felt like sadness and sadness felt like love. The moment the parrot was back in his hand was no different from when he was in the light of bliss.

"Now we must discuss the *other* issue," the Grandmaster continued. "You killed the hawk with a power that we call *empty force*. Empty force is the ability to project your intention and use your Chi to influence objects and people. Empty force can heal or kill; it can be a tool and a weapon. Empty force is attained by disciplined practice or through emotional instability. The most successful students are those who are emotionally unstable but train in disciplined practice. Emotions provide passion and drive you to do the impossible. They can also cause you to escape from reality."

Hunglu looked into the Grandmaster's dark eyes. There was a sense of urgency in them. He had not seen such concern on Moon Over the Water's face ever.

The Grandmaster continued. "Emotionally unstable people escape their pain and try to compensate through magical power. If they develop it spontaneously, they have a great risk of going insane or turning the force against themselves. Do you understand?"

Hunglu was shocked and surprised. Did the Grandmaster mean that he would become insane? Was such a thing possible?

"But *if* emotionally troubled people work through a *disciplined* process, they will resolve their emotional problems through training," the Grandmaster carefully emphasized. "The greater risk to these students is an addiction to power. Unfortunately, students who strictly work through disciplined practice will only be able to use empty force with mixed results; it will be there when they need it, but it is not readily available."

"Your life-review work has stimulated emotions, and the disciplined work you have done has sharpened your focus. Now that you understand and have experienced the power, you will gain control."

"Will I be okay?" Hunglu asked. "Will I be safe from the errors you have seen others make?"

The Grandmaster put his arm around Hunglu's shoulder. "You're safe, Flying Spirit," he said, and they started down the mountain together.

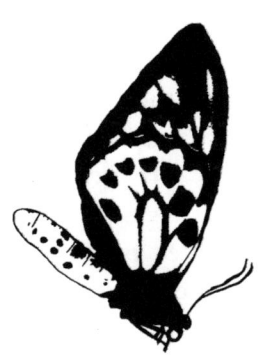

THE GROTTO

The next month passed quietly for Hunglu. He spent his days working with the Tai Chi ruler, practicing forms, and meditating. It was a simple life, almost dreamlike. If it weren't for the parrot, Hunglu would not have known whether he was awake or dreaming.

The parrot was now totally weaned and had become an avid flyer. The incident with the hawk made it aware of predators, so it now always kept Hunglu in its sight. On many afternoons, the bird sat with Hunglu under a tree as the monk meditated . . .

He was flying through space and found himself in a field similar to his father's farm. There was a tree-lined stream running through the wide-open land. It was autumn, the brightly colored leaves almost glistened in the sunlight. Then at the edge of the stream, Hunglu saw a small woman filling a goblet with water. She turned as Hunglu approached and acted surprised to see him. Hunglu tried to greet her but could not speak. The woman was equally perplexed by her own inability to speak.

Looking into her eyes, Hunglu saw his reflection. She was a beautiful woman, very small and fairylike, almost possessing a child's innocence. He felt a peace with her that he had never felt in the presence of any woman, including his own mother. Somehow, he knew her—he had always known her.

Hunglu looked back into her eyes and realized he was truly seeing himself the way she saw him. He knew her thoughts. He could feel her body as if it was his.

It is me, *he thought,* I am her.

The woman moved forward and they became one. Their bodies touched, their souls dissolved into each other. The bliss far exceeded any experience Hunglu had ever had. Then the moment was over and they

133

slipped back into their individual selves. He saw her naked form in front of him, just as he was naked before her. Hunglu looked at her beautiful face and into her eyes and then heard himself speak.

I will find you, he declared. I promise!

Moments later, Hunglu was back under the tree, joy flooding his heart. "I will find you!" he said loudly, "I *must* find you!"

The bird, startled, launched itself from Hunglu's shoulder and flew to a branch above his head.

Hunglu stood up and looked around. He didn't know *who* the woman was or *where* she was, he just knew that if it took the rest of his life, he would locate the extraordinary being he just encountered.

In the morning, Hunglu began his journey down the mountain, eager to find the Grandmaster for counsel regarding his recent meditation. He hurried to the monastery temple, hoping his master would be there.

Hunglu had not been to the temple in so long that it was like a new experience. The statue of Quan Yin was the last thing he really remembered clearly, but today the statue looked lifeless and crude. His spiritual life was now so rich that icons seemed empty and uninspiring. It was with that thought the temple darkened around Hunglu, and he suddenly discovered himself sitting with the Grandmaster in the grotto.

"Where am I?" Hunglu asked.

"At my grotto, of course," the Grandmaster replied.

"But I don't remember walking here," Hunglu said.

"You didn't walk here. Look around you . . . what's missing?"

Hunglu shifted his eyes about; everything seemed as it should be, except something was missing. *The bird.*

"The parrot is with your body, most likely under the tree," the Grandmaster said.

Now it began to make sense to Hunglu. "Yes, yes, of course, I remember now. And you are actually in the temple."

The Grandmaster nodded, confirming his student's perceptions. "What can I do for you?"

Hunglu quickly told the Grandmaster about his meditation and how he was beginning to feel like he was always in a dream.

"Good. This is an important part of your training," the

Grandmaster said. "To realize there is no difference between dreams and reality is essential. As you have concluded, once you know you are in a dream, you have tremendous mastery over all around you. The ruler gives you disciplined control over the levels of consciousness and the power to focus that consciousness on any level you find yourself. What do you think the woman is to you, Flying Spirit?"

Hunglu thought for a moment. "She is important. She is not a guide or a deity; she is in the real world. I believe she is a *real* person, and I met her just like I am meeting you now, outside my physical body."

"Good, continue."

"When we merged, it seemed like we had always been together. Right now nothing seems as important as finding her in real life, and—" Hunglu's mind went blank, as if he could not allow himself to think the unthinkable.

"Go on," the Grandmaster prodded.

"I know I must spend the rest of my life with her, Grandmaster, but—"

As much as Hunglu's heart knew these words to be true, his mind could not accept this fact; he had chosen a life of monastic service. What would he be if he were no longer a monk? His life was pleasant, safe, and predictable. He was focused on spiritual truths, not embroiled in the world of ego and competitions. But now that he had seen this woman, he could not be content living without her.

"You have chosen a different path," the Grandmaster said, finishing Hunglu's thought.

"Perhaps I can still be a monk and be with her?" Hunglu pleadingly suggested.

"Perhaps," the Grandmaster said. "Take little steps to your destination. When the time is right all will be clear to you. We will part ways for now, but I will speak with you soon."

Hunglu returned to his body beneath the tree, where the parrot was grooming his beard.

"At least I know *you're* real," Hunglu said. "Then again, perhaps you're not."

During the next few weeks, Hunglu had glimpses of the woman in his visions but not much more. He was learning a great deal from his out-of-body experiences and met some spiritual friends who were showing him different levels of consciousness. He was also having many realistic dreams in which he was learning about the world. One of his dreamlike experiences caught him completely off guard.

Walking down a path, Hunglu stumbled upon a filthy, decrepit man with scabs covering his body. The man was ill and laying immobile in the dirt.

"Help me to the stream so I can drink," the man begged.

Hunglu saw the seeping scabs and smelled the decaying flesh. He knew that the man could not make it on his own and that he would die without water.

"Yes, I will help you," Hunglu said. Taking a breath, he lifted the man and took him to the water. But as Hunglu carried the man, he realized that he was an immortal soul and nothing could harm him.

The decrepit man gently shifted in Hunglu's arms, and in an incredible metamorphosis, he changed into one of Hunglu's spiritual acquaintances.

"Good! Good! You overcame your fearful illusions," the friend said. "Now you may move forward."

The moment reaffirmed for Hunglu his decision to live a life of service.

Then came a day when Hunglu's life took another drastic turn. He had decided to practice his sword and was feeling particularly powerful when he chose to test the limits of his strength. On a fast lateral swing of the sword, the muscles in his back ripped. He cast the sword off and braced himself for the inevitable.

Incredible pain shot through Hunglu like molton iron, dropping him to his knees. The hideous throbbing injury was amplified even more by his rage at his error. For a long time, he lay upon the ground, cursing himself for being so stupid and arrogant. At the same time he felt so vulnerable, so sad. It would be days until this would heal, and at least a week more before he could adequately defend himself. His only solace was in the knowledge that the injury was not a new problem for him.

Years before, when Hunglu had dropped upon the floor in Lord Chu's headquarters, the impact wrenched his back. That minor strain turned into severe damage when he absorbed the heat and concussion of the bomb blast. The muscle tissue, permanently damaged, caused muscle spasms like the one he was now experiencing. It always happened when his pride pushed him to overtrain.

Hunglu again lay upon his back, looking at the sky and lamenting his foolishness. He was smarter than this. Memories of his painful convalescence at the monastery came back to him. Alone on the mountain, Hunglu felt panic welling up in him. There was no one there to help him. He might die. His mind worked in feverish ways to devise more frightening thoughts.

Finally, Hunglu calmed down and hobbled to his house. Inside, he awkwardly applied an herbal liniment to his back. Though he got immediate relief from the pain, the spasms would take a few days to unwind.

"Some immortal soul I am!" Hunglu scoffed at himself.

Then he reconsidered the error: he had done it to himself by recklessly pushing beyond his limits. Hunglu knew that if he had been patient, he would have performed better over time and *without* injuring himself. After this revelation, even more tension was released from his back.

Hunglu thought about going to visit the Grandmaster, but reconsidered after he took his first step. The pain shot right up his spine, actually making him laugh.

"Oh yes, I'm really going to make it to the Grandmaster's!" he said in a sardonic tone.

Despite the pain and spasms, he knew it was time to make the trip. Hunglu felt a thousand years old as he hobbled down the path, stopping frequently to adjust and rest his back. The parrot was flying with him, so Hunglu knew he wasn't going to wake up from this experience. He slowly shuffled on, not quite sure why he needed to see his master, and was now moving on instinct.

Hunglu arrived at the Grandmaster's cabin only to find another visitor. This was immediately distressing until the Grandmaster quickly invited Hunglu in to meet the guest.

"Flying Spirit, what is wrong?" the Grandmaster asked and then realized, from Hunglu's walk that the young monk had injured his back. "Oh, you are lucky today. Let me present Doctor Han."

The other man rose from the floor and filled the room with both his size and presence. Doctor Han was as big as a bear and had a black beard and dark skin. His head was shaved, which contrasted dramatically with the bushy beard. His eyes were like deep reflecting pools filled with peace. Despite his great size, the doctor's hands were long and thin. Without warning, he reached out to Hunglu.

"Let me fix that for you," Doctor Han said and quickly moved behind the young monk.

Without a second's delay, Han placed two fingers exactly on the spot causing the most pain. The other hand went on Hunglu's abdomen just under the solar plexus. Surprisingly, Hunglu's abdominal muscles felt just as tender as his back. Han gently pushed on the muscles of the abdomen until he found the most tender area, which made Hunglu grimace. The young monk was a little frightened by all the unsolicited touching, especially since Han managed to find all the painful spots without saying a word.

Then there was quiet as Han started to breathe slowly. It felt as though the doctor's hands were moving into his body. Hunglu's muscles were becoming softer and softer, rippling out through his whole body. Suddenly, his back convulsed slightly.

"We're almost done," Han said gently.

All the muscles in Hunglu's back miraculously returned to normal. Then Han touched two fingertips to Hunglu's solar plexus, creating the sensation of a hole being opened; everything under Han's fingers became fluid and loose, making Hunglu sigh, then burp.

"Now I am done!" Han declared with a chuckle.

"Thank you," Hunglu said with great sincerity. Moving his body slowly and cautiously, checking his range of motion, he added, "I feel great. What did you do to me?"

The Grandmaster answered for the wonderful guest: "Doctor Han is a grandmaster of Chi Kung healing, and I think it would be good for you to study with him for a while. That is why he is here."

The doctor nodded his head in affirmation. Hunglu was left speechless but trusted the Grandmaster's guidance to obey without question.

"It is time we all rest," Han said. "We will talk more in the morning."

At dawn, Hunglu, Doctor Han, and the parrot left the monastery and the mountain. Hunglu was quiet during their journey. This was the first time he had been off the mountain since he was brought there eight years before. He noticed a shift in his consciousness; the dreamlike quality of his life had disappeared and he felt normal again. It was not familiar to him to be leaving the sanctuary, and Hunglu was uncomfortable with his emerging feelings. Han, though, kept Hunglu distracted.

As big as Han was, he walked through the woods as silently as a ghost; however, Han was far from a quiet man. The doctor loved to talk and tell stories and laugh. Both Hunglu and the parrot were lured into good humor time and time again by Han's stories. He was indeed a different type of man.

"How did you become a healer?" Hunglu inquired of his companion one day.

"That's a long story," replied Han. "I was the eldest son of a stonecutter and builder. When I was old enough to walk, my father would take me to the quarry and let me watch him cut stones for his buildings. I was playing on scaffolding before I was three, so I learned my father's profession easily. By the time I was an adult, I had become very good at it. Then one day when I was working with two other men high on the scaffolding, something broke, and my friends and I fell thirty feet to the ground. We were killed instantly."

Han laughed, assessing Hunglu's attention; Hunglu did not laugh, he looked at the doctor, mouth agape. Sufficiently content that Hunglu was paying attention, Han continued.

"My heart stopped and I went through a long hallway into a brightly lit room. My two friends were there too, so we made jokes about falling down and started to laugh at what some of the other workers would think about our stupidity for failing to check the scaffolding. Then I noticed some of my ancestors were entering the room. We had a good time talking and sharing stories until bright spirits came and told me that my friends had to go with them. I said goodbye and went off with my own bright spirit.

"My spirit took me to a window and directed me to look out. At first I saw beautiful fields and mountains. Then the world shifted and I saw my whole life. And it was pretty good, Hunglu, which is what the bright spirit said too. He showed me my future and told me that my body was going to be mangled and in pain for years. But he also said I would learn from my pain how to help others heal. I would, he said, become a good doctor.

"I laughed at him. *I'm not smart enough to be a doctor!* I said. *You must have the wrong person.* The bright spirit assured me that I was the right person and that I would learn secret techniques of healing.

He was the one who really talked me into going back. *I am a stonecutter, how am I going to live without being able to use my body?* I asked him. The bright spirit showed me a vision of a little broken child—his back was so twisted and deformed, Hunglu. The vision showed me touching this child in the way I touched you, only for a longer time, and the child straightened out and became normal again. The bright spirit said that this was my destiny. After that, of course I said I would go back. Han suddenly laughed. "I know now that he tricked me!"

"Wasn't there a child?" Hunglu asked.

"No, there was eventually a child exactly like the spirit foretold, but I've since learned that heaven always has more than one way to achieve its plans. If I had said no, some other healer would have been sent to do the job."

"Anyway, after I injured myself it happened that there was a wandering healer nearby, and he touched me and got my heart beating again. I had to lie on my back for months as my bones healed. Everyday I prayed for death. A doctor gave me a lot of herbs and even a small amount of opium, but nothing could really stop the pain. Eventually the bones healed, but I was still very weak—nothing but a bag of bones."

"The healer came back and began to teach me Chi Kung, which made me stronger, but I still couldn't lift my arms over my head. I knew I was finished as a stonecutter. My younger brothers were doing fine, working and helping to run my father's business, but I was just a burden and a source of shame for my family. The next time the healer came through, I left with him."

"The man who healed me was a wandering Taoist master. We traveled together for twenty years, and he taught me all he knew about healing. We eventually became the best of friends. Then one day he said, 'Tomorrow's my day to die, please prepare my funeral pyre.'

I was *shocked*, but I did as he had prepared and instructed me to do. The next day, my master sat in meditation and said goodbye. I sat across from my old friend, holding his hands in mine, and we slipped into a deep, focused state. I could feel his life leaving as I slipped out of my own body. We met on a beautiful mountaintop with stars all around us—even below us.'

140

'*This is the gateway level to the Yin side of human life*', my old master told me. He said there were seven states of being that I could access at this level.

"*When people die*', he said, '*they access the gateway at the fourth level, which is the soul level of being. We are at the third level, the core energy level. At this level we can travel through all dimensions of time and space.*' He told me to stay with him as the levels changed."

"I started feeling lighter and more loved as things all around us changed to pure, bright light. Then my master said, '*Now we will travel through the different levels where souls reside after they die. Each level is for individual learning.*'

"In some levels it was just like in real life, the difference was that unlike earth, every soul on each level was the same. They all had the same beliefs, fears, and goals. Bright spirits guided them, and they saw these spirits not as bright balls of light, but as spiritual leaders that appeared in forms to which the newly dead were most accustomed."

Hunglu hung on every word. He was not even aware of how far they walked since Han began his incredible story. The whole world was disappearing as the doctor spoke.

"There were less and less souls as we continued into the upper levels," Han said. "My master was changing his form as we progressed, becoming more like the bright spirits. Then we finally came to one particular level that was fascinating: on this level, the souls created whatever they wanted. *Oh*, the things they made, Hunglu. There was the *biggest* . . . well, you will just have to see it for yourself when the time comes."

"Anyway, when we reached the seventh level there were very few souls, and they were all bright spheres. The master said, '*This is as far as you can go and still be human. The next levels require a shift to higher forms of being. This is where I'll be staying and learning.*'

"*What will you do here?*" I asked him.

'*Learn from masters on higher levels of being and teach others on the lower levels. Teaching is the most important way to learn. Teaching challenges and fortifies your beliefs. It forces you to organize your knowledge in a manner that conveys the most meaning to your students. But most of all, as a teacher, you learn compassion, patience, and forgiveness. You must be patient and wait for your students to progress, to develop, to understand. You must have compassion for their lives, their beliefs, and their foibles. Once you have practiced patience and compassion for your students' imperfections, then you are able to forgive yourself your own failings. In doing this, you become an even greater source of love. You have taught me more than anyone else, Han. If ever you need to find me, just come back to this place.'*

"I asked him what to do if he was reincarnated but he laughed at me."

'Time doesn't matter, it's all the same dream!' he said. Han paused, remembering the scene. "That's basically it, Hunglu. When I got back to earth, my master's body was dead. I cremated him and spread the ashes so there were no signs of his existence. Then I continued his work."

"Do you ever go to see your old master?" Hunglu asked.

"Oh yes, but not as much as in the past," Han answered. "At first I needed him quite a bit, but as time went on I started to absorb what I needed to know. Of course, there is very little about him that I don't have within me at all times. That is what is called a direct transmission from a master."

"Direct transmission?" Hunglu murmured.

"Yes, this is a concept that you must learn and understand. For example, you know that when two people come together they exchange Chi and consciousness. At a core level they know all about the other person, everything that the other person has learned, the people the other person has been in contact with, and so on. The more you are exposed to a person the more you absorb their knowledge. This permanently alters the way you think and the way your energy fluctuates. If you are in harmony with someone who is more powerful, that exposure makes you stronger, smarter, and more experienced. As you become less resistant to their knowledge, what they know moves forward into your conscious mind."

Hunglu listened carefully. He realized that he was starting to learn many things from the Grandmaster that he was never formally taught, things he couldn't have known from a normal means of learning. Han's teaching was now giving him some insight into that learning.

"However," Han said in a serious tone, "if you are in continuous contact with someone who is negative, or who is not in harmony with the nature of your soul, there becomes an energy conflict." Han smacked his fist against his palm to emphasize his point. "This kind of relationship can make you take a path you are not suited for, and it will eventually disrupt your Chi so much that you become ill with disease."

"Can we learn and be influenced by forces other than words?" Hunglu asked.

"Yes, exactly!" Han replied. "*And* the energy is more powerful. We can ignore words, lessons, and examples, but the energy silently influences our minds. If you stay with me long enough you will know everything that I know and everything that my master and all of his teachers knew."

The two men walked for a long time in silence, Hunglu trying to absorb Han's lessons.

Hunglu asked mostly simple questions to begin with, "How is it that you know where to go on your journeys?"

"The Tao directs me where to turn and how to walk," Han said. "It guides me to where my services are needed. All I need is a clear intention to serve and heal those who will benefit from my services. Generally, the universal god gives me direction in my travels. You see, Hunglu, I am not a physician; I only treat people who need my work, people who are ready to be healed."

Hunglu looked confused. "What do you mean, ready to be healed?" he asked.

"When you injured your back, you came to realize why you hurt yourself, you took responsibility for your part of the injury, and then you made a strong effort to seek out someone to help heal you. When have you ever recovered so quickly and completely?" Han asked.

"Never," Hunglu admitted.

"And why was I at your monastery when you hurt yourself?"

"I think I understand!" Hunglu said happily. "I do understand!"

And he did. Things were beginning to become clear.

As the weeks passed, Hunglu and Han fell into easy, enjoyable patterns of companionship. Each morning they secluded themselves to do their own exercise rituals, each becoming familiar with the other's habits. Then they walked onward, discussing many things. Han began to teach Hunglu, sometimes pointing out medicinal herbs as they walked past various plants. He also pointed out mosses, trees, and animals, then instructed Hunglu in all the details of using and harvesting the natural medicines. The amount of information was, at times, overwhelming. Each day, Han tested Hunglu, and within a few months Hunglu knew nearly two hundred different medicinal preparations.

"You now have learned all the basic preparations that you need to heal most diseases and injuries," Han told Hunglu one day as they walked through a meadow. "The whole earth is a wonderful supply of healing products. Most of what hurts us can be healed with natural remedies found in the areas where we live."

Han opened his arms and turned around in a circle, and Hunglu felt as if he just now woke up to the vibrant splashes of color contained within the field. It was amazing what the universal god made available.

Han continued his instruction. "Knowing how to prepare medicine means you may call yourself a doctor, but you must know more than herbs to be a *healer*. The herbs work on the crude body for short-duration illnesses. But when faced with an illness that doesn't respond to the appropriate herb, you must then look at the Chi of the patient. This is what I do."

"First, determine the vitality of the physical body by how it moves. I know the entire temperament and behaviors of my patients by watching them walk across the room. I know when the Chi force is obstructed by energy or mental inhibitions. Once I've watched a patient walk, I can determine whether the Chi is disrupted by spiritual or mental forces." Han gestured to his body, pounding his chest. "This is not real—you know that from your experiences—yet, it is real and can create great pain. But you, Hunglu, you have felt great pain in a dream, right?"

"Yes, I have."

"So if you feel pain in a dream and feel pain in your body, then where is the pain?"

"In your mind," Hunglu answered confidently.

"*No!*" Han laughed. "The pain is very *real*. It is energy that is used by your mind and spirit to create a living *energy being* within your body. Now, as a healer, you have to discover why the energy being was created. *Why?* Why does this pain or disease exist? The answer is that sometimes the mind and spirit are reacting to bad water or food. Other times the mind and body are reacting to disease from someone else. These are easy to treat with herbs and don't concern me. I am concerned with diseases that the mind and spirit create by themselves, so I watch the body and I listen to what the person has to say about their life."

Hunglu nodded to show he understood.

Han leaned closer to his companion. He was nearly whispering and looked directly into Hunglu's eyes. "A soul will *create* a disease for a positive reason. That reason is to help a person learn to overcome limitations or to terminate the life experience so the soul can focus on another plane of living. When the soul is in control, my friend, there is more peace and acceptance regarding the disease. The patient is fearless and sage-like, living the best possible life under the circumstances. The mind, however, creates diseases for selfish reasons—reasons that usually involve gaining control over the patient's life or even someone else's. Many people are dissatisfied with their lives for various reasons. The mind can create an illness and provide an opportunity for the patient to change their life. People can eliminate the things they don't want to do by having an illness; however, they never seem to know this about themselves. Luckily, they can be tricked into revealing the reasons when they don't expect the questions you ask."

"Mind-created illnesses can also provide an acceptable way to express unwanted emotions. Sometimes people are unable to release the energy of their emotions except through physical illness. For example, anger can cause back pain; sadness can hurt the heart; fear can cripple the legs or destroy the brain. There are many emotions that you will see that create specific diseases. But we must never generalize. Each person is a tapestry with many interconnected threads, and there will always be more than one thread connected to each illness. To find the cause of mind-created illnesses, you must sit and talk with the person over tea. The patient will give you many clues about the origin of their illness by describing their life to you. Look for areas of resistance and unhappiness in their life, and that will lead you to finding the emotions causing problems. There is nothing you can do about a soul-controlled disease other than to provide comfort, but you can treat a mind-created disease if the three requirements of healing are in place."

"What are the requirements," Hunglu asked.

"First, the patient must recognize why they have the disease. Second, they must accept some responsibility for their part in creating the disease. And third, they must make a strong effort to heal the disease themselves." Han made the last statement very seriously, as if it was a code of ethics never to be violated. "People who meet my requirements are the only patients I can heal. They have the power to heal themselves but they need a guide to overcome the resistance created by the mind."

Hunglu listened attentively, mesmerized by Han's presentation.

"Always remember," Han said. "The patient's mind created an energy being within its body that it does not want to get rid of. Both the mind and the energy being have a desire for the illness to survive."

"Can the patient change that?" Hunglu was concerned about living energy beings fighting the healing process.

"Only if the patient demonstrates clear and total intention to be healed by meeting all three of the requirements for healing," Han answered. "But it takes an outside healer to convince the body and mind to release the energy blockage. That's what healers do. They convince negative energy to dissolve and be reabsorbed."

Han's material was again quite beyond his student's reference of experience, but Hunglu was working hard to understand. He had a good knowledge of energy, so he could comprehend how the mind created an energy being within the body. After all, he had killed a hawk with his mind, so it was understandable that someone could turn negative energy upon themselves and die from that experience. But there was an important question Han had not yet answered: "How do you convince the energy to be reabsorbed?" Hunglu asked.

"In the Tao, all things seek harmony with each other. It is natural for things to move toward harmony and love, not toward pain or suffering. Pain and suffering are the result of not knowing, or not choosing, the direction to harmony. I use energy from my infinite soul to touch the obstructed energy. When this congealed, obstructed energy feels the freedom of divine energy, it changes its mind. *I now know freedom*, it says and relaxes its hold on the body before going back to its source. This is the natural order of things."

Hunglu was deeply taken with his new teacher. Han was a reservoir of information. During the past eight years, Hunglu had spent much of his time in silence, effectively isolating himself from interactions with others. He desired nothing more than to be alone with his own thoughts. He had taken pride in his perceptions and conclusions, yet his greatest mentations were mundane in the light of Han's experiences. Hunglu could not get enough of what Han had to say. He had never learned so much in so little time. It made so much sense.

"I was a tadpole in a pond," Hunglu admitted to his teacher, "proudly thinking I knew so much, until I met a frog who knew life outside of the pond. Sharing ideas and life is like the water of a moving stream: it never gets stagnant nor breeds disease."

Han smiled at his student.

Hunglu was also in awe of Han's effortless ability to make the many abstract concepts of Taoism and medicine so easy to understand.

"The nature of Yin and Yang is that everything is interrelated and interdependent," Han taught Hunglu. "You don't know it's light outside until you see dark. As light defines dark, *you* must find out how all things relate to each other. Look around. See how nature moves in balance and harmony. Even the most insignificant action can have great impact. A deer eating an apple in this forest then passing its seeds into the meadow changes the meadow forever. Always look for the smallest relationship you can see."

"If you practice this simple exercise, you will understand the workings of the Tao and, most importantly, the workings of your own mind."

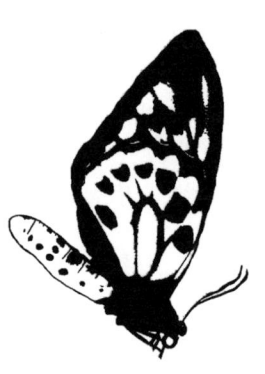

THE OLD MAN

Hunglu began this journey with Han under the Grandmaster's instructions, but now he was beginning to consider a life outside the monastery, a life of healing. A crucial point came when they entered a small village where the herbalist was a long-time friend of Han's.

A frail old man was sitting in front of the pharmacy.

"What's your problem, brother?" Han asked the man.

"My legs are weak, and every day the herbalist massages them for me," the man replied.

"When did this happen?"

"It happened two years ago, and now I can't work in my fields. My sons do all the work, and I feel so useless, especially since my wife died."

"Oh, I'm so sorry for you, my brother," Han said, sitting next to the old man. "When did your wife die?"

"Two and a half years ago," the man answered. "You are a healer, can you help me?"

"Yes, I can. Stand and walk for me."

The old man could barely get to his feet and his walk was a pitiful shuffle that kicked up little clouds of dust as he moved inches at a time. Hunglu looked at Han skeptically. It was unclear why Han so readily said he could help the old man.

"Watch and listen," Han said as he pointed to the man. "See how tense his legs are? They are as rigid as sticks. He is also stiff in his buttocks but loose in the upper body."

"Why do you think you have this problem?" Han asked the old man directly.

The old man looked up with sad eyes. "When my wife died, all the joy left my life. I wasn't interested in my work or anything else. Now I want to play with my grandsons before I die, but I can't," the man anguished.

149

"Let's get you inside and do some work on you," Han said confidently.

As the man hobbled into the pharmacy, Han pulled Hunglu aside. "You see, Hunglu, he has met all three requirements. All of his energy has moved upward and is centered in his head. This takes the energy from the legs. He is also afraid of death, which closes his lower energy center. This will be a good case for you to watch."

Inside, the pharmacy was hot but dry. The walls were lined with desiccated plants, and pottery containing various powders and ointments was stacked neatly on shelves. The light was dim. On one side of the room were several long tables made of bamboo and covered in white cloth. Han laid the man down on one of the herbalist's treatment tables, positioning him on his back. With great care, he touched both of the patient's feet.

The herbalist entered just after the old man was situated. "I learned everything I know about Chi massage from Master Han," the herbalist whispered to Hunglu.

"Come here and hold these feet!" Han commanded, motioning to Hunglu to comply.

Reluctantly, Hunglu grabbed both feet.

"Hold them *lightly*," Han instructed. "Feel for the pulse, not from the heart but from the energy wave going through and around the body."

Hunglu could feel nothing, but continued to hold the feet and tried to focus. After a few minutes, his hands felt as though they slipped into the old man's flesh and suddenly it seemed as though there was a layer of water flowing beneath the skin. The flow was inconsistent.

"Direct your energy wave through his body in the layer you are feeling," Han instructed. "Do you notice what is happening?"

"I don't know what you mean or how to do this," Hunglu said nervously.

"That's all right, your soul knows how to do it," Han assured his student.

Hunglu felt himself pushing energy through the fluidic pulse in the patient's legs. As Han said, Hunglu suddenly understood how to redirect the energy wave. It was a ticklish feeling and Hunglu tried to suppress a laugh.

"It's okay—you may laugh," Han said. "Laughter makes your energy flow better."

"I feel resistance in the knees and lower back and the chest," Hunglu said. "It's like playing with water in a stream; in some places the flow is strong, in others it is weak."

Han agreed with Hunglu's diagnosis, then took over again, touching and poking the man's body in various places. Han spent a long time holding one hand on the man's chest while he touched many points on the man's body with the other hand.

"Now," Han said, "I am releasing the sadness from this man's heart. It has spread roots to many organs and muscles. I am in the process of unraveling all the minor threads so that we can ultimately release the major cause."

Han turned the man on his stomach and positioned Hunglu's hand on the man's tailbone.

In a quiet voice, Han said, "You are touching the two major energy centers of this problem. Our patient has lost control of life and now fears for his survival. Relax your hand like you did in your ruler exercises."

Hunglu did as he was told. He felt tense muscle and bone under his hand. After a few minutes he was shocked to feel the muscle below his hand change into liquid. His hand pushed into the bone, moving deeper. "What am I feeling?" Hunglu asked.

"You are feeling the body of energy created by the mind and spirit that we discussed. It hides and makes you think it is bone and muscle, but it moves the good, healthy body out of position and causes pain, discomfort, and disease."

"Have I changed it?" Hunglu asked, feeling the pulse of a living thing moving beneath the surface of the man's skin. The thought that this energy was a demon also entered his mind.

"You are safe, Flying Spirit," Han comforted. "Remember, in the Tao all things want to achieve harmony with each other. Your calm energy and muscle coaxes the hardened energy to relax and release itself. Now, move your hand softly through the liquid to find what feels like bubbles. When you feel the bubbles, encircle the energy, trap it with your hands, and then relax. It will start to be reabsorbed by the man's mind and soul."

Hunglu did as he was instructed and was amazed at everything that occurred. He felt the energy disappear. Quickly, the whole body beneath him changed. He felt joints moving into different positions, muscles relaxing and elongating.

151

"My body feels like it is being reborn—it's a *miracle!*" the man exclaimed. He giggled with joy as if he were being tickled. "I can feel my feet again."

Han told the man to again lie on his back and asked Hunglu to return to the patient's feet. "Feel the difference?"

Hunglu noticed that every breath the man took moved through his body and down to his feet. Hunglu also felt the man's heartbeat in the feet as well. The energy flow beneath the skin was finally unobstructed.

The man got up with a big smile and moved effortlessly.

"Thank you! Thank you! How can I repay you for this kindness?" the man asked.

"Your smile is enough," Han said.

Happy to have witnessed another of Han's miracles, the herbalist spoke up, "Please join me for tea, master."

Han and Hunglu accepted, and the four men drank and talked for hours. It was a good day, but Han and Hunglu were traveling again by nightfall. The parrot perched safely on Hunglu's shoulder as he walked, and the villagers were amused at the sight of the miracle workers leaving—the bear and the birdman, they called the two Taoists.

Several days later, Hunglu was pushing his ruler during his exercise time when he felt it taking more and more control. His gaze was locked upon the grain's eye as he started losing sensation in his body. At first, Hunglu was hesitant about the feeling, as it was the same sensation he had just before he killed the hawk. That realization made him panic for a moment, but then he calmed, feeling as if he was moving his consciousness into the ball. The ruler was becoming his mind, and when he released his grip the ruler floated between his hands. Wherever Hunglu moved his hands, the ruler levitated in the same location. As his confidence grew, he cautiously dropped his hands to his side. The ruler floated freely before him, and he found he was able to move it with his eyes. Hunglu was pleased and excited but skeptical about what he had achieved.

Han, who had been watching from the bushes, spoke softly: "You have made a great breakthrough, Hunglu. You are now ready to advance further with your training."

Over the next few hours, Han showed Hunglu four more ruler exercises that circulated energy and challenged the mind to maintain the same focus of levitation.

"The eyes are the source of the power." Han said. "But you can move objects with your eyes closed. The physical eyes, when strongly focused upon the object, activate the nonphysical eyes. The difference between the eyes increases visual perception, as if your eyes are moving outside your body."

Hunglu felt exactly what Han was talking about. He could see in many directions at once.

Han continued. "This sensation is often experienced during death—the feeling of moving through a tunnel as the focus moves from the physical to the non-physical. So there really are no *physical* eyes involved. It is the vision of the core-energy self from our shift into the third level of being."

Hunglu remembered Han's experience with his old master, how they had changed levels of being after the master's physical death.

"You say I am using my third level of being to move the ruler in this physical life?" Hunglu asked.

"Exactly," Han answered, pleased with his student's understanding. "Continue practicing this shift of being with your ruler. Then start to use that same state in your other exercises so you can be completely integrated."

Hunglu practiced his new exercises for several weeks before Han attempted to teach him anything new.

One morning, Han began a lecture by saying, "There are thousands of Chi Kung exercises that can be organized in many different ways. They come from many traditions and aspire to many theories. There are fast exercises, slow exercises, and exercises where you don't do anything at all. It is useless to try to memorize the exercises because you will have to adjust them to each individual. You must learn theory and principles instead. The fundamental principle is to remove obstructions of the mind from the body in order to prevent or breakdown the formation of negative energy beings. Don't forget that everything floats in a vast ocean of energy that we call Chi. Every part of us—even the smallest parts of us that we cannot see—float freely, like fish in an ocean. And like those fish, we cannot increase nor decrease the size of the ocean. We can only foul our little place in that ocean with fish dung, and that is what the negative energy beings are, *Chi Dung!*"

Han laughed, as did Hunglu. The ever-aware parrot also let out a short chuckle.

"We open our minds, grab some Chi, mix it with bad ideas, and the waste gets stuck in our bodies," Han explained.

Hunglu was amused by Han's descriptions. "So the Chi Kung *washes* the waste away?"

"Yes," Han replied. "But different ideas and thoughts are stored in different parts of the body. The bad thoughts are categorized by imperative lessons and are stored in hierarchical energy centers, which correspond with the imperatives. The first center is at the base of the spine and controls and stores energy relating to security. This center controls and stores energy relating to our physical security and survival."

Hunglu remembered the old man he had helped Han heal at the pharmacy. The man had obstructions in this area, which were caused by his wife's death and his own fear of death. It had limited his ability to walk and move.

"The second energy center is at the lower part of the spine . . ."

Han spun Hunglu around and put his hand on his sacrum.

"This is the energy center that causes most of the problems. It controls and stores energy related to power and sex." Han smiled. "Life is ever-changing and uncontrollable, but we always try to control our uncontrollable lives—this is why the second energy center is always causing problems."

Han then pointed to his solar plexus.

"The third energy center controls and stores energy for the freedom of the individual self. This energy is related to our impressions of ourselves and our relationships to our peers and society. All your doubts, and criticisms of yourself and others are stored here."

"The fourth energy center is located in the center of the chest, where energy relating to love is controlled and stored. It is also where we store our sadness."

"The fifth energy center is in the neck and throat. This center controls and stores energy relating to justice and equality. Justice comes from truth and integrity, not just in a society, but in each individual. Disease occurs in this center when people deny their truth and do not act according to their soul's imperative."

"The sixth energy center is located between your eyes. This center controls energy relating to intuition and ideas of self-discovery. It helps us to process and understand spiritual information and to integrate it into our lives. Disease comes from ignoring the spiritual influences in our lives."

"The seventh energy center is located at the top of the head and controls the energy of the spirit. Disease is caused when a person resists the spirit or when the person is trying to escape from physical life due to pain."

"The eighth center is the center of the person's whole being—it is the soul itself. This energy center controls our life's purpose and creates our temperament. The eighth center controls our universal energy."

"Hunglu, each energy center controls the body parts and organs within its region. The first center controls the legs and general constitution of the body. The second center controls the sexual organs, excretion, the back, and hips. The third center controls digestion, the gall bladder, pancreas, and stomach. The fourth center controls the heart and lungs. The fifth center controls the throat, teeth, jaw, and thyroid. The sixth center controls the eyes, sinuses, and the brain. The seventh center, like the first, controls the constitution of the body. The eighth center is the controller of all the other centers. The eighth center feeds the vital life force into the other centers. All the centers work together. They must be in harmony with each other and balanced within themselves. Unfortunately this is not normally the case."

Han looked over at Hunglu, but Hunglu said nothing.

"Remember your back injury?" Han asked.

Hunglu couldn't forget it; that was how he had met Han, and since the healing, Hunglu had not even had a minor twitch in his back.

"When I worked on you, I concentrated on your third and second energy centers," Han said, giving Hunglu a lesson he could relate to. "Your injured back was controlled by the second energy center, but it was your self-pride and criticism that drove you to become injured." Hunglu nodded.

"The bomb caused the injury, but your self-criticism over killing those men impeded the second center from healing the wound completely."

Hunglu understood: at the time he was injured he was reviewing emotional events of which he was not proud. To compensate for those poor feelings of self, he had pushed himself hard during his sword practice. The sword had always made him feel powerful, an emotion that he now realized was entirely related to the second energy center.

"My poor feelings disrupted my energy flow," Hunglu said. "And when I added the extra effort, I was hurt."

"Exactly," Han said. "Those interrelationships are what we call *threads*. Threads tie the centers together, tangling and knotting the energy flow. Now let's consider the case of the old man. The man's main problem was the loss of function in his legs. The legs are controlled by the first center, but the problem was much more complicated. The death of his wife disturbed his natural balance of energy. Sadness took hold of his fourth energy center, while his third center was disrupted by his loss of identity caused by his profound sense of loss. His second center was further disrupted by uncontrollable circumstances, while his own mortality and fear of death affected his first center."

Hunglu nodded, remembering the man's suffering and subsequent joy after being treated.

"The threads are what complicated the problem," Han said solemnly. "Sadness, the loss of identity, and a waning desire to regain control of his existence made the man desire death instead of life. Threads from key centers strangled his first energy center, limiting the function of his legs. But once we removed the threads, we were able to treat the real problem center."

Hunglu was gaining a better understanding of the work they had done and the system of healing that Han was teaching him. He wanted to know more.

"Both you and the old man met the three requirements of healing," Han said. "Thus we were able to go directly to the problem and heal it, but this is rarely the case. Most people are unaware of their healing processes. In those cases we prescribe Chi Kung exercises. We prescribe Chi Kung to those who are not yet ready to heal."

This shocked Hunglu, as it was contrary to his teaching and experience.

"Doesn't Chi Kung *stimulate* the flow of Chi through the body?" Hunglu asked.

"Yes," Han answered. "But the body is not real, *remember?*"

"So are the energy flows that I feel when I do Tai Chi and Chi Kung false?"

"No, they are very real," Han replied. "But they are created by the mind, not by the exercise."

Although contrary to Hunglu's education, he now understood that the mind was much more powerful than he had imagined. He had levitated his ruler and killed a hawk with empty force. He had released an energy obstruction created by fear and sadness in a man who desperately needed help. These things were beyond Hunglu's comprehension before his training—now they had become his reality.

"So how *does* Chi Kung work?" Hunglu asked.

"Chi Kung exercises the body in the energy centers," Han explained. "It stimulates the energy centers, forcing the mind to reconsider all the stored emotions and bad decisions. Only then will the mind start to meet the three requirements for healing . . ."

Hunglu was beginning to feel as if he were becoming synchronized with Han's mind and added, "The body stimulates the energy center that governs it, putting pressure on the mind to change its course."

"*Yes!*" Han said. "And the daily practice fortifies the intention to get well, meeting two of the three requirements of healing. So prescribing a Chi Kung exercise requires that you understand the energy center that is causing the problem and use an exercise that will stimulate that part of the body. Chi Kung should be prescribed to ensure that all the centers are equally balanced. The eighth center also needs to be stimulated by exercises such as holding the ball. A good set of exercises will prevent the development of disease in a reasonably healthy person. Temperament, however, determines where the energy obstructions will occur, so you must always prescribe Chi Kung exercises to match the person's temperament rather than prescribe from a particular tradition. The exercises you choose should eliminate the tension from the body and unbalanced parts of the mind. Choose an exercise that matches both the person's mind and relaxes the body. If these two principles are observed the mind will be balanced and release tensions that restrict the body and Chi."

"Is that the secret of immortality, Han?" Hunglu was now coming to the realization that the body wasn't real, and immortality, in his mind, was all that was left.

"You are close," Han answered. "True immortals are pure spirits who present themselves in human form. They are illusions who are given physical attributes by those who see them. On the other hand, there are physical immortals who are humans and have lived well beyond normal lifespans. They have eliminated obstructions between the mind and soul, keeping them in harmony and making them immune to aging and diseases."

Suddenly a thought occurred to Hunglu: "Han, how old are you?" Han laughed. "One hundred and seventy-seven years this spring."

Although surprised by Han's answer, Hunglu did not doubt that it was true.

"But I'm a baby," Han chuckled. "My old master was over two hundred and fifty years old."

"Why did he die?" Hunglu asked.

"Every living thing dies," Han replied. "I live because I *enjoy* being human. I also serve a purpose as a teacher and healer. But a day will come when my soul will want to work on the nonphysical planes and I will leave. So it was with my master."

"Life is a game, but it's not a game that is won by how long you live. It is won by how well you learn and serve. First, serve the gods and the Tao, then serve your fellow man."

The months passed easily for Hunglu. He steeped himself in his training and listened for hours as Han provided him with insightful advice necessary to master the healing arts. It was wonderful to have a companion such as Han, and in many ways Hunglu felt that they developed a relationship like brothers—a realization that made Hunglu understand how much he still yearned for family.

Han trained Hunglu to prescribe Chi Kung, prepare herbs, and do hands-on healing. He sought out larger towns and cities to provide many opportunities for Hunglu to practice his new skills. Han believed, as did most masters, that a student needed to practice on a thousand patients before they could begin to even know their craft.

At the same time, Hunglu was beginning to get exposure to life beyond the monastery. He spent hours listening to the life stories of his patients and came to realize that Han was correct: people and illnesses could be classified by temperament. Hunglu learned to read people's temperaments by how they walked, sat, stood, and even breathed. The patterns were clearly illustrated in all patients, regardless of their wealth or education.

Aside from building his own experience, Hunglu watched and learned from Master Han. He observed Han heal the disfigured and even raise a child from the dead. But, surprisingly, Han refused to treat far more people than he helped. 'This one is a soul problem' or

'This one is not ready to heal,' he would say. Hunglu learned that very few sick people met all three requirements for healing, and Han was religious about not making exceptions.

Within two years, Hunglu developed great skills as a healer. He truly enjoyed the process of helping others become well and loved the people he worked on. The more he practiced healing, the more his heart opened. Hunglu started to lose the boundaries between himself and his patients. He could feel their bodies, understand their minds, and even look into their past or future for clues to their well-being or lack thereof. Hunglu had become a kind, compassionate, mystical healer. He was happy with himself.

Then one day Hunglu felt himself being yanked from his body during an intense meditation. In front of him was a very bright spirit he immediately recognized as Han.

"It's time for you to begin your education on other, deeper levels," Han said. "Follow me."

Han drifted up and Hunglu followed. They went to a small house where a family had gathered. An older woman with very white skin and hair lay on a nearby bed. Relatives were bidding the old woman farewell. Their love for her was clear by their level of grief, which Hunglu felt resonating through his being. He could feel their sorrow and their thoughts. As he floated above the room, Hunglu realized the woman could see him clearly.

She smiled at him and spoke to her family. "The good spirits are here to take me home!" she exclaimed.

The others did not know what to make of the old woman's statement and whispered to each other about delirium.

"Yes, little sister, we've come to take you home," Han said. "Prepare yourself and your loved ones."

The woman then spoke personally to each member of her family, recalling shared pleasantries and exchanging blessings. The relatives seemed relieved by the old woman's unexpected lucidity. It was as if she were suddenly energized by her death.

"Goodbye . . ." she said, expelling her last breath.

It took a moment before the old woman's spirit began to leave her body. Hunglu didn't know what to expect and looked at Han for guidance.

"Don't be concerned." Han smiled. "Your soul knows what to do." As the woman's spirit rose from her body, the room around them disappeared, and they hovered above the corpse. The old woman's relatives were grieving, but the woman herself was free from her pain and physical limits.

The three spiritual forms moved upward. Reality changed around them, reshaping itself into a bright, golden tunnel around the woman. Hunglu and Han could still see her through the translucent, ethereal layer separating the two planes of existence. The woman smiled and appeared to be growing younger as she moved forward. Hunglu and Han traveled along outside, watching. Later, Hunglu would find himself thinking of the experience and feel a great joy in his heart. It was almost as if they were watching a cocooned butterfly transform into a thing of golden beauty.

"The tunnel is the result of the shifting of the mind from one reality to another," Han explained. "We are merely observers of her constructions."

When the woman moved out of the tunnel, relatives greeted her. A husband who had died long before was there to embrace the woman and the two of them talked for a long time. Hunglu did not see the form of a man; instead, he saw a wavering, shimmering being of light.

"This being is a higher evolution of the husband's soul," Han said, explaining the differences between their perceptions. "His soul exists at many levels at once. The highest level is always the first to meet the departed. The woman will see him as she desires to, not as he truly is."

Hunglu changed his perception and reached out to the woman's mind to see what she saw. Through her consciousness he witnessed how she transformed reality to become more comfortable with her beliefs—the man was young and handsome. He felt tremendous love and compassion watching the woman's life review. The more he saw, the more his compassion for the woman grew. Hunglu's light expanded, and he started to lose his self-identity, becoming himself a brilliant being of light.

"What's happening to me?" Hunglu asked.

"You are changing your level of being," Han responded. "Trust your soul, it will guide you."

Hunglu followed Han's advice and found himself absorbing the woman into himself as they were both transported to a higher level of being. Almost immediately they came to a pastoral setting, where two bright spirits were waiting. The woman drifted to them and disappeared. Their connection was severed.

Hunglu slowly moved back into his body and was humbled that a mere mortal, such as he, could be so much more. Though he did not fully grasp what had happened, he would soon learn that the woman's rapturous transformation had simply been the unleashing of the goodness that was already in her.

For a month Hunglu continued guiding departed souls to their destinations. At first Han led the trips, then other spirits assisted until, finally, Hunglu could act alone.

"You have done very well and learned most of the dimensions of the Yin side of life," Han said one day. "Now you must learn how a soul can change its state of being, no matter what level it is on.

There are seven levels of being that each human soul can access. The first level is the state of normal everyday awareness in our physical lives. It is using all of our senses and living a full, human experience.

"The second level of being is the state of mind that we achieve when we do Kung Fu, Tai Chi, Chi Kung, light meditation, dream, and allow our spirit to travel out of our bodies. After death, some souls stay at the second level of being to further evolve in human energy forms. They repeat lives in physical and nonphysical reality over and over again, learning as they go.

The third level of being is when the mind moves its awareness beyond the physical body into its core energetic self. From this state of being, all levels of human existence and guidance can be accessed. This is the level where most spiritual training occurs, in both the Yin and Yang sides of life."

Han gazed out into the distance, as if looking through time, then he continued.

"The third level of being is how most people enter death, though most of them will then drop into the second level of being before going on. Others progress to the fourth level of being, which is the soul level. This is the level of core divine love, of divine bliss, but the individual mind still exists to give humans meaning to what is happening. In death, most people meet guides on the third level of being. Then a guide uses compassion and acceptance in their soul to open their companion's heart moving them to the fourth level of being. Only then can the soul express the divine love within it, radiating it outward to all within its presence. Most people believe this love comes from the guides. But it is actually internal to each individual's soul. Generally, a person's mind has no human references to this feeling, so it says, *The guide gave me the greatest love I've ever felt!"*

Hunglu had also believed that the guide provided the intense feelings of love until he became a guide himself. In fact, he was frightened by the adoration he had received from some of the souls he encountered.

"Each soul contains this divine love," Han continued. "Once a person accesses the pathway to this love, it can never close. A person can open this path through death or a large spiritual ritual involving many people or meditation rituals. Everyone should try to move into this level of being as often as possible."

Hunglu realized that Han was always fully at the fourth level of being, and this was the secret of his longevity—the soul controlled his life without interference from the mind. Han was perceived by most souls as a saint. No one questioned or opposed him, nor did *he* oppose others. It was simple harmony between minds. Even wild animals would seek out his presence: once, while Han was practicing his Chi Kung, a leopard walked into camp and lay down to watch. The leopard purred and rolled until Han was finished, and then it left.

Hunglu remembered thinking, *This is the true power of the Tao. No sword or bomb was as powerful as Han's love.* It was a great blessing to know someone at the fourth level of being.

"It is difficult to maintain the fourth level of being," Han continued. "Most who reach the fourth level drop back to the third, and very few living people are able to hold the fourth level of being for more than a few minutes. But that's when miracles occur. Healings are most successful when both the healer and the patient are at the fourth level of being at the same time. It is truly wonderful when this occurs.

"The fifth level of being is our evolved guide-self. At this level our soul is complete. At the fifth level we have all the knowledge we have gathered through our lifetimes, combined with the knowledge and experiences of our twin soul."

Hunglu gave Han a quizzical look, letting his teacher know that he did not understand.

Han explained carefully. "Each soul divides into twin parts that enter into their own life experiences. One part experiences the Yin aspects of physical life, while the other experiences the Yang. They each go through multiple evolutions and gender changes. Ultimately, the Yin and Yang rejoin at the fifth level of being to guide and teach. To sustain the fifth level and become an immortal who can teach on both sides of life, we must rejoin with our twin soul."

"How do twin souls rejoin?" Hunglu asked.

"We are always joined on the fifth level of being. But to rejoin and sustain the fifth level requires that we meet and bond with our twin soul in the human experience."

"Have you met your twin soul?" Hunglu asked.

"Yes, I have," Han said with a warm smile. "I started seeing her in dreams at first. Then, as my meditation evolved, I started accessing my fifth level of being. The more I experienced the fifth level of being, the more I became familiar and accustomed to my twin soul's spirit. Then I started actively seeking her out. We joined eight hundred and eighty years from now."

"*What?*" Hunglu exclaimed.

Han laughed at Hunglu's incredulous surprise.

"The Tao is a great ocean in which all that ever was and ever will be floats," Han explained. "Each life ever lived, by *your* soul or another, can be experienced as easily as reading a scroll. I merely sought out and lived the life where our souls joined."

"Where is she now?" Hunglu asked.

"She is living a life as a servant in the lands to the north and west of here, a land that was stolen from the sea. She has yellow hair and gray-blue eyes."

Both Han and Hunglu were amused by the thought of a yellow-haired woman.

"Once you bond to your twin soul," Han said, "you always know where the other half is."

"You have actually lived in a future lifetime?" Hunglu asked, astonished.

Han's memories put him in a softer, almost transcendent disposition as he explained. "Each life is a dream, Hunglu. When you are within the dream you forget everything that exists outside the dream. So if we review what you've already learned, you'll have a better understanding of how we travel into another lifetime."

"Now remember, most people exist in the first level of being during the day and move to the second level of being while they sleep. They move back and forth this way, learning and evolving until one day they move to the second level and slip into the third by dying. Since they can't sustain the third level, they move back into the second level, now believing they are at the first level. Do you understand me so far?"

"Yes," Hunglu replied.

"They learn what they need to know for their next life experience, and then they move into a *new* first-level life. They continue this process until they learn to access and use the third level of being."

"The soul continues to evolve by discovering the fourth level of being. Once the soul has been rediscovered, all the individual lives start a quest for a spiritual reunion. The person starts to more actively explore the Yin side of life until the barriers between the two sides of life are very thin. Then the soul starts to access its fifth-level self, learning to become a guide and teacher for others. The fifth-level being has direct control over its lower-level evolutions. The fifth-level self also knows all the lifetimes of the twin souls and can guide them to achieve its needs. The fifth-level being is a spiritual immortal."

Han paused, letting Hunglu digest this information.

"Once I was able to sustain the fourth-level state of being it was very easy to access knowledge and experience and live my life through it."

Hunglu admitted his confusion and asked Han to explain more carefully. Han drew a circle on the ground and put eight little stones in it. He then counted out four of the stones to Hunglu.

"This stone is your first level, this is your second, this is your third, this is your fourth," he said, identifying the purpose of each stone. "The other four stones are your twin-soul's levels. All of the stones are independent, but they all are within the circle of the fifth level. Eight is the basic unit of the *I Ching* and the immortal soul."

Hunglu knew the influence of the *I Ching* in all of Han's teachings about the spiritual levels. "So as I understand you," he said, "I am an immortal soul who has many levels of development within me." He picked up the stone that Han had pointed out as his third-level being.

"But I am only operating at this level. Still, I can access my fifth-level self at any time and find my twin soul."

Han smiled and nodded.

"When I meet my twin soul and we join, will I *then* be able to sustain my fifth level of being?"

"Exactly! You're becoming so smart." Han patted Hunglu's shoulder and continued with his lecture. "The sixth level of being is when thousands of complete souls unite to share consciousness. This level of knowledge is staggering to comprehend. When you access your sixth-level being, you are omnipotent. You know all things that have and will ever happen in the human experience. Now, understand that the sixth-level being governs humans according to their imperatives. Souls that share the same imperative are mates which have the same basic purpose. They also have many ways to express their purpose. We have an infinite number of soul mates to help us with our purpose, as friends, guides, and lovers all working toward the same sixth-level purpose—a purpose that is so grand we cannot know it."

This news excited Hunglu. He wanted to know what was beyond the sixth level of being, but there Han became enigmatic.

"The seventh level of being is completely beyond our comprehension," Han said, his arms gesturing outward to show how big the seventh level was. "It is when sixth-level beings combine with others beyond our universe. We can experience this union at our level but never quite understand what has happened to us. We are far more than we can ever understand or accurately imagine. A tadpole can understand what life may be like outside the pond, but even then, he cannot imagine what your parrot sees and experiences within the sky."

The two men, teacher and student, looked around them. The night sky was above the hills surrounding their small camp. An infinite number of stars filled the heavens, glittering and dancing, each distant but seemingly within the grasp of a determined mind.

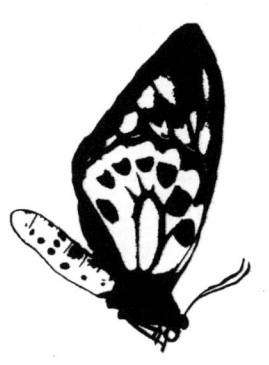

THE GUIDE

Sometimes Hunglu would stop and consider all he had learned from Han. The immensity of his training was, at times, overwhelming, yet Han was a careful teacher who never forced too much on Hunglu during any one lesson. The knowledge Hunglu had acquired was a product of years spent in training and practice. But lately Hunglu was thinking more and more about his twin soul. He had been seeing a woman more in his dreams, the same one with whom he bonded years earlier. Each day, Hunglu felt the compulsion to find her.

Along the extensive journey, the parrot had matured and become incredibly agile in flight. It would no longer have much to fear in the way of hawks. Hunglu liked to throw pine nuts in the air and let the parrot catch them. It was a fun trick that he taught the bird by accident one morning when he dropped a nut and the bird, swooping by, caught it. Then he started throwing nuts to the bird. Watching his parrot's acrobatics, Hunglu knew that finding his soul mate would be like catching a nut in the air—he would have to grab her as she flew by. There would be one chance, and it might come when he least expected it. He paid close attention to his dreams, waiting for that moment.

Hunglu was drifting among the stars with a guide. He saw a mass of people—dull gray shapes—marching to a cave in a grotto. On either side of the cave was a guard. Walking aimlessly into the cave, the people disappeared one after another. It seemed to Hunglu that the cave had a pulling force to it, drawing the people in against their will.

"What is this?" Hunglu asked the guide.

"This is the entry point back into human life," the guide responded.

Without understanding why, Hunglu felt afraid. It was like watching people march to an execution. He quickly shifted to the soul level, where he felt an overwhelming love and sadness for the poor spirits entering new lives. But moving into the fifth level of being, everything changed. The people transformed into a rainbow of light flowing into a shimmering pond. The rainbow changed shapes and speed, undulating in mesmerizing patterns. The guards turned into spiritual light beings, guiding with love and monitoring the fluctuations of the never-ending pattern.

Hunglu rose above the light and saw his parrot flying toward a small house in the forest. The bird had never appeared in any of his dream travels before and Hunglu was unsure of the meaning of this image. Outside the house was the girl—Hunglu's twin soul—picking herbs in a garden. The parrot landed on her shoulder. She petted it and went back to picking the herbs. Then the bird flew up into a tree and waited on a branch. Hunglu focused on the parrot and realized it wasn't his bird after all.

The dream unexpectedly shattered around him and Hunglu sat up so quickly that he frightened the parrot. It squawked violently and hopped up and down on its perch.

"I'm sorry, little one," Hunglu said as he stroked its feathers, soothing both it and himself back to sleep. The bird in his dream—what could it mean? The night wore on under a brilliant moon, but his dreams were empty.

MASTERY

"We have to leave for the southwest today," Han said after he and Hunglu concluded their morning exercises.

Hunglu was quiet for several hours, but as they walked through a forest, he felt an unexpected question welling up in him. "How do we reconcile our religious practice and beliefs with what we have learned through our adventures?"

"This is a question that is not a question, Flying Spirit," Han answered. "If you only had wondrous experiences in your life, what would you believe about life and death?"

"I don't know what I would believe," Hunglu said. "I have always altered my Taoist beliefs to be in harmony with my experiences."

"*Ahhhh*. You adjusted your religion to meet your beliefs," Han said, grinning. "Everyone creates their religion around their experiences, but it is like Tai Chi forms: you must do the movements that are hard for you so you may develop the skills you would not have if you were allowed to do whatever you wished. Religion, Hunglu, is most important. It helps us to develop a moral code, personal discipline, and integrity. The experiences that we know as true teach us how we are one with all things. Religion also teaches us how to be kind to each other and how to apply truths in a world filled with limitations and emotions. For those who are operating on the first and second levels of being, religion is the only message available to point them to something more than their individual survival. It provides them with prayers and rituals that will alter their awareness and program their minds to attain the third level of being."

Hunglu remembered the many times he was in the temple praying, losing track of time, and feeling an exquisite sense of awareness expand beyond his body. He remembered the peace he found by having clearly defined rules and how he had to discipline himself to meet the rules.

"I can understand this," Hunglu said. "My training made me a better man."

"This is good," Han said. "It is now our purpose to help others find truth and comfort in whatever they believe. From our perspective, we have no position so we can only offer support and confirmation of others' beliefs with our knowledge and experience."

"But what if their beliefs are wrong?" Hunglu asked with sincere concern."

"But is there such a thing as *wrong* at the sixth level of being?" Han pressed.

Hunglu considered that at the fifth and sixth level of being everything was in perfect harmony and moving at its own pace. "No, nothing is wrong at those levels," he said. "The challenge, then, is to accept and see the natural order of what is happening as perfect."

"Exactly," Han replied proudly. "And now you can consider yourself a master."

Hunglu was stunned into disbelief. "*Thank you*, Master Han," he said humbly.

Hunglu quickly recognized the great honor Han just bestowed upon him. Old Taoists didn't believe in permanence; to be a master one had to live it. There were no physical icons to prove mastery; when one became a master it shined like a light—it was a reflection of the way one lived life. Han's comment meant that Hunglu was living every moment as a master.

"Han, I don't see everything as perfect," Hunglu said sheepishly, aware of his lack of mastery.

"Of course not," Han agreed. "To achieve this acceptance you must be operating in your fourth level of being."

"So when you are working from your soul, you will always see perfection?"

"Yes."

"Then I'd better start practicing," Hunglu said urgently.

The two monks had wandered near the outskirts of a village. The landscape looked familiar to Hunglu, but he had been so many places that he saw similarities in every village. Han pointed to one of the homes nestled against a hill and they went to it. When the two monks knocked on the bamboo door, an old woman answered, obviously surprised to see her unexpected guests.

"We've come to help you," Han said.

They went with the old woman into the house and found a small boy about six years old lying on a mat. His mother was by his side and helped the boy sit up. He was weak from pneumonia and crippled in the left leg. His brown eyes had lost their glitter and his mouth hung open, gasping. Shadows filled the small home and the air was ripe with the smell of sickness.

Han turned to Hunglu and whispered, "This is a good case for you."

Hunglu slowly knelt down and examined the boy. He placed his hands upon the child and scanned the youth's energy. There was a lung problem brought on by a lack of will to survive. Hunglu changed his level of being to the fourth level and saw the child's past; the boy had fallen into an irrigation ditch and broken his leg. The bones healed wrong, crippling the boy, and that was when he lost his will to live. The child was ill equipped to deal with both the pain of a poorly healed leg and the shame of his disfigurement. He could never be the heir to his father's farm.

Han spoke to Hunglu in a quiet voice: "A trained martial artist learns to focus his blows with his intention. That intention creates an energy that enters into the body of his victim and can become a permanent part of the victim's body and mind. The same is true from energy delivered by an accident. The victim's fear can be so great that the mind freezes the energy of the accident into the body, causing the body to become permanently crippled. Because this is an innocent child, you can treat his soul and it will heal his other problems."

Hunglu positioned himself over the boy, placing his hand on the center of the small chest. He changed his level of being to the fourth level and entered the small child's body with his consciousness. Within his mind's eye, Hunglu saw the soul of the boy as a shimmering sphere of light. As he had done in so many death experiences, Hunglu opened his patient's heart and expanded his soul to embrace the boy's soul. The two souls harmonized and Hunglu noticed a familiar sensation that he could not explain as he reached out and touched the boy's crippled leg exactly at the point of injury.

The mother, who had been holding the boy's hand while Hunglu did his work, could not see the activity that was happening in the other dimension. She only saw Hunglu touch her child's leg and watched as the boy quivered. The child's breathing paused for a moment then returned to normal, the sound of congestion quickly dissipating. The mother sat in astonishment as the boy's breathing continued to regulate. Then she gasped as the child's leg straightened after months of being bent at a grotesque angle.

Having just performed his first miracle healing, Hunglu was as shocked, excited, and terrified as the grandmother and mother. He carefully helped the child to his feet.

The boy hugged Hunglu with uncontrollable love. "Thank you so much, Uncle, I will go show my father!" he said and went out the door, calling for his father to come see him.

"Please, monk," the mother urged, "come see my husband. He will want to thank you in person."

Before Hunglu could say anything, Han spoke "My friend will be glad to go with you." Leaning over and whispering in Hunglu's ear, Han added, "I will meet you on the north side of the village. Take your time."

Hunglu was stunned into immobility.

"Go!" Han laughed. "*Go!*"

Hunglu trotted off after the mother and boy. As he jogged through the village, his eye caught the sight of a well at the center of the village. Suddenly he froze, his heart anxiously pounding. It was the well where he had been plucked from certain death so many years before. *He was home.*

"Come, come!" the mother called after him.

Hunglu, his mind locked on the image of the well, hurried behind the woman. Ahead, a man stood at the edge of a field and looked with disbelief at his once crippled son running towards him. Then the man glanced at Hunglu. There was something about the face, the eyes: the man was, Hunglu knew, his brother. The two of them moved slowly toward each other. Hunglu could see tears of joy in his brother's eyes.

"I don't know how to thank you!" The man paused and looked at Hunglu. "Do I *know* you, monk?"

"I'm your brother," Hunglu said with tears welling up in his own eyes. My name is Hunglu."

Brother embraced brother, without hesitation.

Night in the village came with the sweet sounds and smells of celebration. There was feast and nearly every citizen came to greet Hunglu and welcome him home. Some of the older villagers remembered him and his family, but most of them did not talk much about Hunglu's family in the years after his mother passed away. Not a word was ever mentioned about Sunyin, but much was made of Hunglu's father.

The parrot fluttered in and about the rafts of the farmhouse, mesmerizing children and adults alike. There was food and music, then the inevitable dwindling of guests as the evening wore on. Hunglu, exhausted, found himself a place on the clean floor to lay out his blanket, despite his brother's protest to sleep in the kang. The reunited family was soon asleep and the village became silent. A sense of peace filled the small valley, for one of their own, a special man of many talents, had come home and performed a miracle.

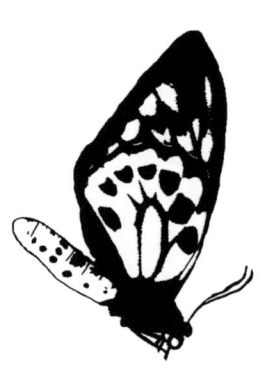

THE LESSONS

The villagers expected Hunglu to remain with them and there was a feeling in the air that grand things would happen. This was not to be, though. Despite his feelings of having finally come home, Hunglu knew that he was not destined to remain in the village, for he had not yet encountered his soul mate. He left amid many protests, but assured the villagers that he would return one day. They attempted to give him many gifts, but Hunglu declined.

"But I will always carry your love," he told them.

It was the following afternoon when Hunglu reconnected with Han outside the village.

"It's good to see you again," Han said. He was hunched over a small fire and warming his hands.

"I'm sorry I was gone so long." Hunglu smiled at his old friend, happy to be with him again.

"You and I have shared a lot of life," Han said with a knowing smile. "There is nothing else I can teach you now. You're free to stay here if you wish."

Hunglu laughed. "You have one hundred and seventy-seven years of knowledge to teach me. I am not ready to leave you now. I know I'll come back here to visit, but I need to return to the monastery first."

"Then I will make that journey with you," Han said. "I'm no longer content to travel alone."

For years, the monks had been traveling roughly in the direction of the setting sun. Now they turned around and began their long trip east to the monastery, healing and lecturing disciples along the way.

Over the many months they spent on their journey, Hunglu concentrated his meditations on finding his twin soul. When he connected with his fourth level of being he often got visions of her. In this way, he discovered that his soul mate was an herbalist healer living somewhere in China. He could see all the details of her life, but could not discern her name or where she lived.

"Don't worry, you'll find her," Han assured him as they traveled. "You both must be ready for each other before you can meet. I had many opportunities to meet my twin soul in my future. We crossed paths *three times* and just missed each other. I was searching for her and she was searching for me, but we both had more things to learn and goals to accomplish in our lives before we could meet. Those lessons and accomplishments proved to be pivotal in making our relationship work. Separately, we developed the skills we needed to accomplish our group purpose."

"What lessons did you learn, Han?" Hunglu asked.

"Oh, the most important lessons," Han replied. "I learned about the polarity of relationships and the nature of god and all the spirits."

Hunglu knew how important this was. "Well," he said, "*tell* me about them."

"To understand relationships, you must first understand the nature of Yin and Yang, otherwise you will always have bad relationships . . ." Han removed a coin from his pouch and held it up for Hunglu to see. "Most people wrongly think that Yin and Yang are opposites—they are not. It is similar to how this coin has two different sides, one plain and one with engraving. One side could be considered Yang and the other Yin, but both sides together create the coin. If you remove one side you no longer have anything."

"Yes," Hunglu said as he smiled, "but what about light and dark? Surely those are opposites?"

"Close your eyes," Han directed.

Hunglu, though surprised by the request, did as he was instructed.

"Do you see me?" Han asked.

"No."

"Am I still here?"

Hunglu, knowing Han, thought the question was probably a trick but still answered with what was obvious: "Yes!"

"Now open your eyes."

Hunglu did as he was told.

Han was smiling. "Just because you cannot see light in the

darkness doesn't mean it's not there," he said. "Some animals, like cats, can see clearly in light, like us, but also in the darkness. So there must always be some light for them to see."

Hunglu, having spent many a night walking through the forest, understood what Han was saying.

"There is always a little Yin in Yang, and a little Yang in Yin," Han explained. He held up another coin, pointing at a square hole in the middle.

"Even the *nothingness* of the hole requires the *something* of the coin in order to exist. Do you understand?"

Hunglu nodded.

"The process of life will always have us entering into relationships that are unbalanced and unproductive from our perspective. However, a love relationship should always aspire to the highest level of balance and productivity. Each person has an internal spiritual longing to be whole with the source. Love is a union, a complete desire to bond with the object of our affection. It is man's destiny and his *purpose* to love. You need to understand that every loving relationship has a Yin and Yang nature. One partner is the active Yang and the other is the *reactive* Yin. There is a natural drive to select a partner who has a compatible polarity—not a polarity of opposition, mind you, but a complementary polarity, a polarity that is strong where we are weak. Our mate should be of the same soul imperative, a soul mate who is governed by the same sixth level of being and one who is naturally of similar temperament."

"When soul mates combine, Hunglu, there will be differences in temperament that are created by upbringings in different families and cultures. This variance in life paths and upbringing will bring together complementary ideas and skills, but at the core level, the soul mates' temperaments are the same. It is in this manner that the deepest, most intimate levels of bonding and communication can occur. We see the world in the same way and from the same source as our soul mate."

"Unfortunately, this is not how relationships normally go for most people. Generally, people operate at their first, second, and fledgling third levels of being. People at these levels are preoccupied with physical life and being because they have not yet connected with their fourth level of being, their soul self. When we operate at these levels, our mind tricks us into selecting an opposite polarity imperative rather than a complementary polarity soul mate."

Han looked at Hunglu's attentive but slightly perplexed expression. "This is a little confusing," Han admitted, "but very important."

"Why do we select a complete opposite for a soul mate?" Hunglu asked.

Han grinned. "A person who hasn't done a life review to understand their inner motives or discover their core temperament is living a life based on how they have been taught to live by their families, village, and culture. They make choices based upon who they think they are rather than who they *know* they are. This creates an internal conflict between thinking and knowing, and they begin to criticize their own shortcomings."

Hunglu already understood how internal criticism had limited his perceptions of who he was and how much he discovered about his truth as he did the life review. He felt lighter in mind and body after his review. Reminding himself of this, he was ready to learn more.

And Han pressed on. "When we feel below the standards of ourselves or our society, we seek out mates that compensate for the shortcomings for which we have been criticized. An individualistic, selfish power imperative will select an open, bonding, love imperative for a mate. An organized, quiet, security imperative will select a fun-loving freedom imperative. A rigid justice imperative will choose an excessively liberal humanitarian. A grounded mechanistic progressive will choose an ethereal universal imperative. Each is trying to become whole through the other. They admire and revere the attributes of their polarity. The greater the individual self-disgust, the greater the polarity difference between mates. But the goal is to discover the self through the polar self, and the mates act like polishing stones, grinding against each other until a gem is created." Before continuing, Han shook his head, recalling the difficulty and pain of the process. "Some partners work to change because they think they are broken. They want to develop, to achieve their full potential and make their relationship successful. These are the Yang partners. Meanwhile, the Yin partners do nothing because they define themselves as not being Yang. They *resist* the Yang effort to grow at every turn, changing only as a reaction to the changes of the Yang partners. Yet this is not true for people who are of the same temperament and nature."

"How do the imperatives resist each other?" Hunglu asked, trying to understand the complex dynamic Han was explaining.

Han wrinkled his brow in thought. "A person whose imperative is power will abuse a person whose imperative is love. The love imperatives make all their decisions based upon the love they will give or receive. The power imperatives make all their decisions by what they can control and gain. For example, the love imperatives look at art as beauty, while the power imperatives look at art as a possession and a symbol of power. The two live in very different realities.

"However, if the polarity between the partners is not too great, they will exchange ideas and talents and build and develop each other. If, though, the extremes are great, both partners will close their hearts and develop disease as a means to either gain control or exit the relationship. There are so many unhappy people in the world today and almost all of that unhappiness is caused by lack of love. Hunglu, everyone wants to love and wants to feel loved, but they don't succeed. They fail not because of a lack of skill or ability to love but because of poor choices in *who* they love. Poor decision-making skills then get passed down from parents to children, like the inheritance of a water buffalo. Eventually, a whole world can't find love. Take, for example, how a cat and a mouse can live together by suppressing their instincts and nature in order to live in harmony and flourish with each other. But a cat can't *love* a mouse in the way a mouse can, nor can a mouse ever meet the needs of a cat—except as *lunch*. Seriously, though, neither one can ever have a fulfilling, loving relationship with the other as long as they both have to suppress parts of their nature to be with each other. Ultimately, they will lose themselves and die. The soul becomes so overpowered by the emptiness of the relationship, it has no choice but to terminate the life experience."

"Now, the fourth-level being is one who lives in the soul, and the soul contains boundless expressions of love. Every soul, no matter what its imperative, lives to love, for that is what every soul is . . . *love*. As a mouse must find love from a mouse, we have to find a soul mate to have true love. There are millions of soul mates for each of us; all we have to do is reflect upon who we are and we will find someone just like us. Sadly, most choose not to discover who they are. They lack the courage to face their emotions and fears, and the result is that they select whoever is there and suffer without hope of finding true fulfillment. Really, how can you find love if you can't find yourself?"

Hunglu shrugged his shoulders. What Han was saying made good sense to him, and the ideas further inspired Hunglu to push on in his quest to find his soul mate.

"A person who doesn't see himself and honor and love himself certainly cannot love a twin soul." Han looked directly into Hunglu's eyes. "You have done your review, you have felt your soul, you have experienced divine love, but only human love can heal the wounds of a human heart. You know that spiritual love enables you to know your nature and to love yourself at the divine level. But this is only a shield to protect you when seeking out human love. Be careful and do not hide like most spiritual seekers do. Hiding in a monastery and feeling blissful is no different than being an opium addict. It takes courage to love, to face hurtful feelings, and even when you *do* find your twin soul, it will not be easy, Hunglu. You will still have fear, you will still be insecure with yourself, and you will hurt each other's feelings. On the other hand, a good relationship will polish you into a gem, it will allow you to shed unwanted emotions and thoughts and be at peace . . . You will feel as if you are *home* when you are in your soul mate's arms."

"I will tell you that long ago I discovered how the Yin and Yang relationship applied to god as well. We know the Tao has intelligence, that it does things for a reason and purpose. It is universal, permeating all things without a human consciousness. This is the Yin of god," Han declared boldly. "The Yin of god naturally creates a Yang god— a god that has a personal human nature. There are millions of people who believe in a single personal god with whom they can communicate, and one that behaves like a person. For centuries this has existed, and it will still exist long into the future. With so many minds focusing upon this belief, humans create it as a truth as easily as they create disease in their bodies. You, Hunglu, have seen the power of the mind and know this is true. People created an individual god, a god that we can use and communicate with. A god that we can draw power from. A god that can heal the evil in the world."

"Would this be the same with any deity?" Hunglu asked suddenly.

"Exactly," Han replied. "All religions have saints and sub-deities to perform certain tasks. They *really* do."

"Then it is important to honor these deities as real and harmonize with their power?" Hunglu suggested.

Han nodded. "Yes, because the focus upon a positive force for good prevents minds from creating evil. The power of religion to muster masses of people to focus on positive prayer, positive deities, disciplining their behavior, and doing truly compassionate acts can offset all the unfocused negative thoughts in the world."

Hunglu stopped walking and looked directly in Han's eyes. "If this can do so much good, then fear and negative thoughts would act the same as in the body, creating disease in society, right?"

Han was very pleased with Hunglu's powers of deduction, and it was clear to him that Hunglu had reached the critical mass of knowledge that produced mastery. There was just a little more work to do. "However," Han said, "sometimes good is evil."

"What do you mean?" Hunglu asked.

"When fear causes people to focus upon doing actions to prevent a war or disaster, that fear actually starts to create the war or disaster. Each act of prevention inspired by fear is actually like a prayer for a disaster to occur. In time this fear becomes a part of the culture and creates strange illnesses within the population."

Hunglu considered Han's theory. "If a person feared an illness and they religiously practiced Chi Kung and took herbs to prevent the illness, the fear itself would still be developing an energy being within the body. The efforts would prevent the illness but, in turn, create a new and different illness. So how do we stop this sort of problem?"

"I just go to the moment when the seed of fear is placed and stop it from growing in my patients," Han answered. "It is our purpose to move through time, to access lives, and provide the knowledge others need to stop their misguided beliefs. We inspire people with new ideas they have never considered. In one future time I lived in, people possessed bombs that could destroy cities larger than Nanking. They could poison the air and water for hundreds of miles around the destruction. They had tools to talk to people anywhere in the world as easy as we are talking to each other now."

Hunglu struggled to imagine the type of world Han was describing, but concrete visions eluded him.

"The people in the future become so smart that they no longer believe in the gods or anything outside of what man can produce or understand. There are sad times in the distant future. Everyone will mistrust each other and focus upon fears. This creates more wars and diseases until humans are left with nothing to believe in. Their ability to understand will fail them, and their pride prevents them from using their religions. That was why I was there. My twin soul and I, along with millions like us, were sent to live in this period to guide and offer options to those filled with fear. Our message was simple, but the task difficult. We were meant to teach people to ignore the illusions and fears around them, to go inside themselves and find their souls. We didn't have to reach every person, though; each person who moved to a third level of being had the capability to influence a thousand people with their energy. Each fourth-level being might influence a million or more. In the future, there will be a beautiful healing. Small teams, like my wife and I, will work on unraveling individual threads woven in the tapestry of fear. We will focus on selected students, knowing that their energy can convince others to evolve."

Hunglu was captivated (and concerned) by Han's description of the future.

"The immortals will appear in physical reality to work miracles and train people to rise to the fourth level. But their real work shall be on the Yin side of life. The immortals will reveal the Yin to their soul mates, and this will happen through meditation and death experiences, providing others new options to their fear by letting them experience divine love."

"Does it work?" Hunglu asked.

"Yes, it works: after thirty years that world changes. The population begins to accept spiritual principles of divine love in everyday life. Of course, that is the easy part. People will still want to run away from life and into spiritual love. They won't want to do life reviews or discipline their minds and bodies and change the negative patterns in their lives. They want only magic and bliss. Yet, they eventually learn that there is no difference between Yin and Yang, that heaven resides within the balance of the two dimensions of reality. The two must be integrated."

"How is this done?" Hunglu asked.

"Through the soul." Han placed his open hand on his chest. "All we need to do is move into our fourth level of being. Then we exist in harmony on both the Yin and Yang sides of life. Of course, this is not easy. The mind and body must be integrated through disciplined practice in order to transcend their limits." Hunglu listened intently.

"Your ruler practice integrated your mind and body, disciplined your mental focus, and opened the gateway to the true potential of human existence. The practice made you shed unproductive thoughts and habits and discover subtle patterns of living. This placed you into the third level of being with full integrity."

Hunglu nodded.

"Your healing practice has opened your heart to love. You share and connect to all manner of people. You truly experienced the oneness of all people and things. You opened your heart to love yourself through loving others. The open heart allowed you to fully integrate with your soul and the fourth level of being. This created greater awareness and allowed you to completely explore and experience the Yin side of life. Now, my friend, you are ready to explore more dimensions of connection and love than you can imagine. In the future you will teach others, through *many* different methods, what you achieved through your ruler practice. The future is where I first meet you, Flying Spirit, not our past."

Hunglu knew in that moment what Han said was truth. Yes, they had met in the distant future, and though the details were vague, somewhere in the depths of Hunglu's unconsciousness, he recognized his friend from another time and place.

"Our work here directly influences the success of our work in the future," Han said, laying his hands on Hunglu's shoulders. "We must work in the present to change the future."

Hunglu considered that the whole model of the Tao was based upon interconnected oneness. Only the immortals would have enough perspective to see the consequences of human actions and provide appropriate guidance. The benevolent intervention by an immortal was an act of love that permeated all levels of beings through all times, and the greatest gift an immortal gave was their guidance. His purpose in life became clear to Hunglu at that moment.

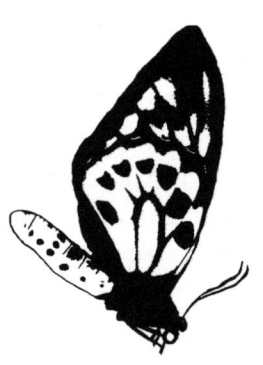

REUNION

Hunglu felt himself floating through space to the shrine of the Butterfly Immortal. The Immortal changed his level of being so that he appeared as pure energy. Hunglu changed his level of being, too, and became the Butterfly Immortal. At that moment, he was complete. He instantaneously rediscovered all of his lives and everything he needed to know to sustain a fourth-level state of being. He saw himself continuing upon the path of a healer, just as he was trained to do. He understood why he would have to leave the monastery, but he also knew he would never be alone again.

Near the end of their journey, Han could see changes taking place in Hunglu. The young monk was developing a peace and completeness about him, a glow.

"What did you learn in your dreams?" Han asked one morning when Hunglu seemed particularly happy.

"I learned that *I* am the Butterfly Immortal. I learned that I am complete and that I will accomplish all the things I need to do. *I am not alone.*"

"It is a glorious day," Han said.

Hunglu now understood everything. He was full of energy and bursting with joyous plans. Until he could sustain the fifth level of his being Hunglu had the gift of the Butterfly Immortal's counsel, guidance, and intervention. He turned to Han and said, "I know that you and I are eternal friends whose hearts will always be linked. I also know where my soul mate is, and though it isn't time for us to be together yet, our paths will cross soon."

"This is very good!" Han exclaimed.

Hunglu traveled only a few more weeks with Han until, at last, they reached the monastery where their friendship began.

"Thank you, my dear friend, for all you have given me," Hunglu said. "I will miss our talks together."

"And so will I," Han agreed. "Maybe *I'll* find a bird to keep me company."

At the monastery gates the two men embraced, their minds spilling over with memories of the adventures they had been on together. The years they had spent on their journey now seemed like only moments. Then they separated. Han walked off to another destiny, and Hunglu re-entered the place that first changed his life.

The monks greeted him and there was a feast prepared by Old Cook. This time, Hunglu did not hide or act shy around his brothers, he desired to be with each of them, to share with them his stories of spiritual enlightenment.

Hunglu spent the next month talking with the Grandmaster and others. During that time he gave away all of his possessions to his brothers in the monastery. One day he removed his robes and put on clothes of a common man; he would always be a Taoist, but he no longer needed external markers to prove it.

Hunglu meant to continue being a wandering healer for the time being. He would return many times to the monastery to visit his friends and his path would occasionally cross with Han, on *both* sides of life. He had one final journey to make.

HOME

On a cool autumn afternoon, Hunglu was walking down a path in the forest. In the distance he could hear the rustling of a stream around the bend. He whistled for his parrot, and the bird came down from the trees above.

"We will stop and have a drink ahead, little one," Hunglu said.

As they reached the bend, the parrot suddenly lifted off Hunglu's shoulder and disappeared into the brightly colored leaves above. Hunglu looked up, and whistled again. This time the parrot did not come to him. He waited for a long while, then called out, "I am leaving without you, blue friend!"

He heard the parrot squawk farther down the trail. Hunglu hurried toward the sound.

As he ran around the bend in the trail, Hunglu suddenly saw a woman standing by the water. When she turned, it was clear that she recognized him, just like in a dream. Hunglu knew that he had at long last found his soul mate, and she looked even more beautiful in person.

"Hello, Flying Spirit," the beautiful creature said in a sweet melodic voice.

"Hello, Little Bird," Hunglu responded back. "I have been searching for you."

Behind them, the young couple heard a pair of shrieks and hoots. They both looked up to see their parrots preening each other. Then Hunglu and Little Bird embraced each other in a welcoming hug that transcended lifetimes, for they knew they were both *home!*

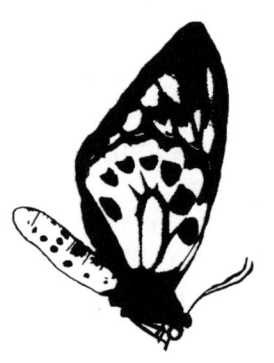

Check out our website at www.whitewillowtaichi.com for more information about our school, products and history.

Your thoughts and comments are also appreciated. You can contact us at:

White Willow Publishing
7433 Montgomery Road
Cincinnati, OH 45236

e-mail: vince@whitewillowtaichi.com
Telephone: (513) 791-9428